Severe and Profound Brain Injury

Severe and Profound Brain Injury is a comprehensive guide offering clinicians practical tools, techniques, and ways to structure thinking in approaching how to best assess and provide neurorehabilitation to patients with the most overwhelming and complex neuro-disability. Advances in acute care will lead to increasing numbers of people surviving with complex neuro-disability and more families will be challenged by a confusing and devastating form of loss. Most clinicians will not have encountered this level of impairment in clinical practice and can feel deskilled, challenged by how best to help, and overpowered by the questions it raises.

This book proposes a paradigm shift in how to assess and formulate the cognitive, behavioural, and emotional difficulties in complex neuro-disability. The task for clinicians is to look for ability in the face of global impairment, rather than focus on areas of disability. Practical advice is provided on how to approach thinking about the issues and design bespoke, person-centred assessments from first principles with robust methodology. Prolonged disorders of consciousness and locked in syndrome are discussed in detail. Guidance is given to keeping the person at the centre of decision-making and intervention planning, particularly as so many will lack mental capacity and require best interests' decisions to be made on their behalf.

This is essential reading for established clinicians wanting to develop expertise working with these patients and their families, clinical psychologists, neuropsychologists, other health professionals, students, and trainees.

Sonja Soeterik is a consultant clinical psychologist (UK) and a registered clinical neuropsychologist (NZ). She has led specialist complex neuro-disability services both in the community and inpatient settings. Her interests include working with so-called hard to assess people and complex mental capacity decision-making.

Sal Connolly is a consultant clinical neuropsychologist who has led and developed specialist services in nationally and internationally recognised centres for people with brain injury. Her interests include working with the teams around people with complex neuro-disability including their children, families, and multi-professional teams.

Sarah Crawford is a consultant clinical neuropsychologist and is currently the Professional Lead for Clinical Psychology and the Lead Clinician for mental capacity at the Royal Hospital for Neuro-disability. Her research interests include mood, cognition, and communication in severe and profound brain injury.

Severe and Profound Brain Injury

A Clinician's Guide to Complex Neuro-Disability

Sonja Soeterik, Sal Connolly and Sarah Crawford

Routledge
Taylor & Francis Group

LONDON AND NEW YORK

Designed cover image: getty images via Calysta Images

First published 2026
by Routledge
4 Park Square, Milton Park, Abingdon, Oxon OX14 4RN

and by Routledge
605 Third Avenue, New York, NY 10158

Routledge is an imprint of the Taylor & Francis Group, an informa business

British Library Cataloguing-in-Publication Data
A catalogue record for this book is available from the British Library

ISBN: 9781032665962 (hbk)
ISBN: 9781032665931 (pbk)
ISBN: 9781032665986 (ebk)

DOI: 10.4324/9781032665986

Typeset in Optima
by Newgen Publishing UK

Contents

Acknowledgements

We are acutely aware that we only enter peoples lives during the worst chapter of their life, when they have survived, against the odds, the most extreme brain changes and everything is unrecognisable to the life they led before. We meet their families at a time when they are facing great uncertainty and are contemplating time defined by 'before' and 'after' the brain injury. We want to thank the clients and families, who even when facing such great challenges and pain have been teachers and guides into the world of complex neuro-disability, and our many skilled colleagues who have shared and taught us so much from their experiences. We want to specifically mention Professor J. Graham Beaumont who has mentored, advised, and been so influential in our careers and our thinking about the contribution of neuropsychology with this clinical population. Thank you all for shaping our work.

Finally, a special acknowledgement to our own families who have supported and facilitated the preparation of this book.

1 An introduction and reflection on the challenges of working with adults with catastrophic brain injury

Brain injuries can create fundamental life-long changes. Whilst there is a shared language to describe the severity of an insult to the brain at the time of injury, there is much less commonality in accurately describing the longer-term outcomes of a brain injury. Catastrophic and profound, complex neuro-disability encompasses a cohort of people with very severe *outcomes* following a brain injury. These severe consequences encompass a separate construct from that of the initial insult to the brain (Rose et al., 2023). There has been a recent tendency, particularly in medicolegal and independent clinical practice settings, to use words such as 'catastrophic' or 'devastating' to describe some severe brain injuries, particularly when life will be very different for the person in the future. However, these terms have been applied indiscriminately to any injury with life-changing outcomes, including spinal injuries and amputations. These words therefore do not exclusively refer to the clinical population we are addressing in this book, and the consequence is a lack of shared language between professionals to describe it. When you want to highlight this cohort of people who have survived a severe brain injury but are left with a life that is fundamentally unrecognisable from how most people would consider 'living' to look like, with global impairments and the most severe, devastating, catastrophic, and profound outcomes seen in complex neuro-disability, the words unfortunately have lost their power to adequately describe it.

Current classification systems group these people in either 'Severe Disability' or 'Vegetative State' categories of the Glasgow Outcome Scale-Extended (GOSE; Jennett et al., 1981), and as people who require Complex Specialised Rehabilitation and care, using The Rehabilitation Complexity Scale-extended (e-RCS; Turner-Stokes et al., 2012). However, although potentially categorised in the same broad group, these patients can present with significant differences in presentation from each other. The box illustrates common characteristics of people with catastrophic, severe, and complex neuro-disability outcomes in order to illustrate where these differences can occur:

DOI: 10.4324/9781032665986-1

Common characteristics of people with catastrophic and complex severe neuro-disability

- Documented significant insult to the brain and likely polytrauma.
- May have had conservative management of neurological injury in acute phase OR may have had significant neurosurgical interventions in attempts to reduce secondary damage to the brain (e.g. removal of brain tissue, insertion of drains within the brain)
- Person may be missing part of their skull (burr holes, be without the bone flap, have titanium, or ceramic skull replacements) and at risk of falls and further injury
- Positional management needs; most likely bedbound, and attempts are underway to seat them in wheelchairs and build up their seating tolerance
- Experiencing physical changes e.g. contractures, tight muscles (spasticity) or flaccid limbs requiring splinting, botox, medications, and tendon releases
- Requiring 24-hour care and full assistance with personal care and all activities of daily living
- May have swallowing problems requiring clinically assisted nutrition and hydration (CANH) typically through a feeding tube placed in their abdomen (PEG or JEG) which is also used to deliver medications
- May have difficulties managing their own saliva
- Airway management needs, possibly needing a tracheostomy tube to assist their breathing and support for suctioning
- Be doubly incontinent of urine and faeces
- Acute medical status may fluctuate (e.g. chest infections, PEG site infections, urinary tract infections)
- High-level nursing care needs to maintain tissue viability; at risk of developing pressure sores
- Epilepsy
- Communication impairments
- Sensory impairments
- Cognitive impairments – likely to be described as cognitively 'unassessable'
- May exhibit some challenging behaviour
- Specialised equipment needs requiring specialist beds and mattresses, specialist seating systems, specialist showering trolleys, and specialist splinting
- Require a large multi-professional team

There is a range of diagnostic descriptions of people who might be described by these characteristics. These include:

- Prolonged disorders of consciousness (PDOC)
- Vegetative state/unresponsive wakefulness syndrome
- Minimally conscious state
- Locked in syndrome
- Severe neuro-disability
- Emerged from PDOC
- Significant, severe, profound, catastrophic, or devastating brain injury

This severe and profound outcome after a brain injury is essentially unrecognisable from a person's preinjury functioning. There are multiple and global impairments in sensory abilities, communication, cognition, and physical abilities. The question 'how has this injury affected the person?' is far less relevant than the question of 'what, if anything, can this person now do?'. The overwhelming nature of the disabilities is so obvious that combined with the invasive and intrusive nature of care that is likely to be required for life, this level of complex and profound injury severity regularly provokes questions for families, professionals, and wider society alike about the moral, ethical, philosophical, spiritual, and legal implications. We often hear reflections and musing such as

> *Is this really living?*
> *What if it was someone you loved?*
> *What would you want if this was you?*
> *Would it have been better if they died?*
> *Do they know who I am?*
> *Why them?*
> *How could God allow this?*
> *Isn't it barbaric to keep him alive like this?*
> *What if she gains a little but not a lot and can realise how bad things are, won't that be worse?*
> *I hope they don't know what is going on.*
> *No one knows what is possible only God.*

For some cultures, it is wrong to even ask or think about these questions, and the valuing of the sanctity of life is paramount, something bigger than humans and only for a God. For others, it can feel futile to provide treatments without the expectation of significant neurological recovery. This dilemma of having the physical presence of the body of the loved one but without their psychological presence has been termed ambiguous loss (Boss, 2000) and is described as one of the most complex forms of grief to cope with, as it creates a limbo and the need to have a goodbye without the person then actually physically leaving. For some, it remains important to provide physical care and contact to the body whilst behaving as if the essence of the person is still there (Cipolletta et al., 2016).

The evidence base for survivors of such complex brain injury is very limited, partly because this clinical population is largely excluded from research studies due to their inability to provide informed consent and the heterogeneity of their presentations. Whilst this diversity creates challenges for research, it also creates challenges for clinical practice and evidence-based neurorehabilitation. It is common to hear that the complexity overwhelms staff. Patients are described as 'unassessable' and staff feel deskilled in how to approach their work with them. We have often lamented that there was no good book to give to assistants, trainee psychologists, and qualified staff from psychology and other disciplines to help them conceptualise the work. Writing this book is our attempt to fill this gap. It stems from years of thought-provoking discussions, providing direction and advice to others in clinical meetings and supervisions. Therefore, we have written this book not as a summary of the literature or a critique of it, but as a set of guiding principles and practical steps to approach working with people with complex neurodisability – a way to think about the problem(s).

We want to highlight the importance of having clinical supervision from someone who has experience working with people with complex neurodisability. We have repeatedly seen evidence of people whose experience is with less severely impaired people with brain injuries making assumptions and offering advice that is well-intentioned but unhelpful because they lack the right frame of reference or the confidence to test out what might be considered 'unusual' or 'unstandardised' therapeutic approaches. Some of these assumptions are discussed later in this chapter. However, the result is often that they reach for the 'recipe book', e.g. the bag of standardised tests or a manual for therapy. We see psychologists taking a deep breath and trying to do weekly sessions of talking therapy with someone who they have assumed must be depressed but who lacks the cognitive abilities to engage with or benefit from therapy, to the extent that it is questionable whether they have the cognitive foundations to be depressed at all. We see people saying someone is 'not assessable' at all or, conversely, creating a 'bespoke assessment' but one that does not have proper rigour and cannot provide evidence for the results the psychologist claims it shows. This is largely a reflection of a lack of experience with this patient group and the differences that are required, which necessitates the mentorship of someone who has built these skills.

Whilst a brain injury can occur at any point in a person's life, this book focuses on people who have acquired neurological injuries as adults and who are now in neurorehabilitation. Many of the considerations and techniques outlined may have relevance to other clinical populations such as children and adolescents with brain injuries, people with profound learning disabilities, and adults with progressive neurological disorders. However, injury as an adult creates a unique set of expectations about what a 'good recovery' looks like and a return to a level of baseline preinjury functioning and premorbid personality that is desired by families. There is clearly a difference in perspective between families who have known someone for a long time prior to the injury and hence see them in one light (as a much cherished member of their family) and the professionals who enter their life post-injury and start from the point of significant and complex neuro-disability (hence primarily seeing the disability to manage). In clinical practice, it is not uncommon to find families' perceptions of the model of recovery centred around what professionals will 'do to' and 'do with' the person that will promote change. Yet amongst professionals, the mechanism of change is often viewed through a lens of 'disability management', a process of stabilising and optimising a person physically, medically, and environmentally in order to enable the brain to recover as much as possible and establish the best assessment conditions to examine underlying functioning. The disability management and any active rehabilitation possible happen in conjunction. However, this creates a dichotomy from the beginning, a family idea that change in functioning happens through professionals' direct intervention, and a professionals' model that they are setting the scene to encourage, enable, and optimise natural recovery. Clearly, there is a window where these two sets of ideas converge and interact, but when professionals consider that 'disability management' and any active rehabilitation have been achieved, but the family can see the person has not recovered, this has the potential to create periods of great distress and conflict between professionals and families. It can also be a point where families look outside the medical model and seek to consider alternative models of healing and well-being to experiment with.

In our experience, this patient group often has problematic assumptions develop. This is not an exhaustive list but an illustration of things that commonly occur:

1 *Locked in.* Perhaps one of the most common assumptions and deepest fear is the idea that the person is somehow able to understand what is happening but thus far has not been able to show or communicate that. There is often a belief that erroneously evolves that the apparent level of externally visible disability is not mirrored cognitively and that the person is in fact locked in their body in some way. This may be associated with a belief that the person's brain has somehow inadvertently been put on 'pause' or 'standby', and that the right visitor, conversation, activity, music, or memory being provoked will enable them to transcend from this place and re-enter normal life again. This is the so-called 'sleeping beauty' belief, that the right stimulus will transform the brain-injured person back to who they were, and it is often portrayed in movies and television in this way too. This leads to a series of behaviours from families to attempt to find the missing key to unlock recovery. This can form part of families' ideas about what rehabilitation is and what it should be trying to do. We have seen a similar phenomenon amongst experienced professionals who are

diligent and caring, and who are anxious about not 'missing' something or not having sufficient personalised materials to find the right 'hook' to help pull the person into recovery. The motivation of both sets of rehabilitation providers (the professionals and the family members) is to maximise the functioning and recovery of the person, yet at times the different approaches can seem to be at odds with each other, for example, with professionals trying to control sensory overload and cognitive fatigue by reducing sound, lighting, and movement to enable the brain to rest, and the family being lively and noisy, trying to make something interesting and exciting in the hope of eliciting a response.

2 *Over-reading into a minimal response:* When the person can do so little, any indicators of ability can be cues to families that the person is really still present. For example, a familiar characteristic of the person like an eyebrow raise can be interpreted by families as indicative of greater underlying cognition, communicating dismissive intent, or perhaps a humorous response. If, and when, people improve a little more and are able to exhibit a greater range of responding, it can often be easier for everyone to better understand the underlying impairments, as it is possible to demonstrate their difficulties such that everyone can see and agree on them.

3 *Choice Making:* In the face of so much impairment and disability, both families and professionals search for signs and indicators of any ability. For example, if it is observed that the person appears to be able to show a response to mean 'yes' or 'no' in relation to something in the environment, like wanting the radio turned off, this can quickly get extrapolated into an assumption that the person is able to use this technique to answer more complex and abstract questions. Beliefs can then evolve that a person is capable of understanding 'everything'. Careful assessment is needed to establish the reliability of such apparent choice-making and determine if it is true for basic, concrete, here, and now choice-making, versus more complex and abstract choices. This will be discussed in later chapters.

4 *Techniques and skills used to assess other populations with brain injury can just be simply modified for this cohort of people.* In reality, an entirely different approach is needed for people with catastrophic brain injury outcomes. It's not the same as assessing someone who has a difficulty in only one area. For example, if someone is blind, but all other sensory, communicative, and physical abilities are intact, then you simply carry out a standardised assessment without using visual stimuli; if someone is deaf but all other abilities are intact, then you carry out your usual assessment without using auditory stimuli; if someone's sensory abilities and speech are intact but they cannot use their arms and hands, then you carry out your standardised assessment using verbal and visual stimuli but with no motor demands. In contrast, this population rarely has standardised testing designed for their needs, and their domains of impairment are far more widespread.

5 *Explanations and assumptions evolve:* Due to their profound and complex neuro-disability, many will struggle to understand what is required of them or be able to initiate a response. They may lack the motor planning or skills to enact a response, have delayed speed of processing to absorb and respond etc. Some professionals and families may observe this lack of responding and develop their own explanations for it. Family explanations are commonly generated from their past experiences with the person and understanding of their 'normal' preinjury personality and characteristics, the existing knowledge bases they hold, and in the age of the internet, their 'google search'. This means flawed attributions are often posited as psychological explanations (she is 'depressed') and motivational explanations (he's 'not interested') or concerns about the abilities of the person before compared to the simplicity of the request ('she was at university, this is too easy for her so she won't do it').

6 *Maintaining hope when world assumptions have been shattered.* Many families and some professionals will share concerns about the complexities of human cognition and the limits of science and medicine in understanding it. People were often not expected to survive the initial injury and have already transcended expectations provided to families in the early acute stages. This sets up ideas about the intrinsic ability of the person to recover on their own as they have 'defied' received medical wisdom to date and are clearly a 'fighter'. This can feed into beliefs that there is so much unknown that reliance on health care professionals' opinions is unwise, especially in the context of the acute providers having been incorrect already. With the availability of the internet, families may do a lot of their own research in trying to make sense of the person's presentation and seeking to ensure that all possible and helpful approaches are being trialed and nothing is being missed. It is not unusual to meet people who have conducted searches online but have been unable to avoid common pitfalls of doing this without sufficient background knowledge, e.g. they may conflate different conditions (such as conflating coma recovery with Vegetative State recovery) and then develop expectations about their family member based on an inaccurate aetiology (such as stroke versus traumatic brain injury in PDOC). When recovery is not proceeding at the rate hoped for, families may search for alternative therapies either by researching experimental treatments on the internet, or by seeking solutions through complementary techniques (such as Reiki, craniosacral therapy, acupuncture, aromatherapy, or massage). In these situations, teams should consider these requests in line with best interests decision-making principles under the Mental Capacity Act (2005), taking particular care of any physiological risks such as triggering pain, hypersensitivity, or vertigo.

In the past, professionals would rarely encounter people with catastrophic and complex neuro-disability, even those professionals specialising in inpatient neurorehabilitation. This was in part due to the fact that in some countries the ability to get people to acute specialist medical care quickly, within the 'golden hour', would impact their chance of survival. Cultural differences in the facilities available and pragmatism of decision-making in the 'Window for Death' (Kitzinger & Kitzinger, 2013) would limit how long people critically unwell were maintained. In other countries after stabilisation, people would be discharged home into the care of family, and the complexities of nursing someone with such complex needs without a large team, specialist equipment, and access to urgent medical care would be life-limiting. Since advancements in the provision of defibrillators in public places, in emergency and acute medicine in general, and the development of specialist hyperacute stroke units and Major Trauma Centres in the United Kingdom, survival rates for adults with acquired brain injuries have increased by approximately 50% (or 500 people per year since 2010) (All Parliamentary Group on Acquired Brain Injury, 2018). Whilst not all these people will have severe brain injury outcomes, it does mean that there has been an increase in people surviving with catastrophic and complex neuro-disability. In addition to more people surviving severe brain injuries, advances in equipment (such as airflow pressure management mattresses, CANH), the ability to manage comorbidities and complications, and medical and nursing care have meant people who do survive are also living longer with catastrophic and complex neuro-disability. This is illustrated in the description of Russell below. Internationally, some countries have legal provisions for euthanasia and societal acceptance of following the expressly, stated wishes about how a person would want to live if they acquired a catastrophic and complex neuro-disability (for example the Netherlands, Switzerland, Austria); in other countries, the requirement to provide assessment, rehabilitation, care, and support is expected. This means professionals who may have never, or rarely, encountered this clinical group previously are now more likely to, and a paradigm shift in thinking is required about how to best approach this work.

Russell was involved in a road traffic accident whilst riding his bicycle to work. He was trapped under a lorry, and the Helicopter Emergency Medical Services (HEMS) attended him at the scene assessing his initial Glasgow Coma Scale to have been 5/15. He was intubated and sedated, and the first responders performed several life-saving techniques.

On transfer to the major trauma centre, he was assessed to have complex polytrauma (rib fractures, open book pelvic fractures, skull fractures, torn organs, extensive bleeding, and haemodynamically unstable), and extensive traumatic brain injury (DAI, SAH, SDH, herniation). He required emergency surgery and neurosurgical intervention to perform a craniectomy, insert an ICP bolt, and subsequently a VP shunt. A tube for CANH was inserted. He acquired a range of infections in intensive care including Covid-19. He had a number of seizures.

Once sedation was weaned, his eyes were open but he did not follow commands or attempt to communicate.

Russell's wife Johanna and daughters who were at university, kept a steady presence beside his bed while he was in intensive care. They were clear that he had a strong faith, had always insisted that life was sacred, and would have wanted all treatments possible. They massaged his legs, played his favourite music, held his hand, and talked to him continually. A visiting rota of friends and family was developed along with a Facebook page giving daily updates to everyone about his progress and sharing photos of him. They advocated strongly that he would want to see the family dog and attempted to reunite Russell with things that had strong personal relevance and salience.

Russell continued to lack the mental capacity to make decisions about his care and treatment, and referrals were made in his best interests to a Level 1 neurorehabilitation unit to assess and manage his condition. It is at this point that clinicians who work with high levels of complex neuro-disability will first meet Russell and begin to explore his abilities.

Underpinning our interest in working in complex neuro-disability is working out what to do when you cannot do what you were initially trained to do. This is not a clinical population that enables you to (a) talk to the person and gain insights through their self-report, (b) administer standardised tests to gain understandings of their cognitive strengths and areas of new difficulty, (c) observe them and quickly develop data to draw hypotheses from, (d) take a good history to understand how their preinjury experiences in life could well be impacting their current presentation, (e) be able to rely on your well established clinical models to understand patient presentations like for depression or anxiety in the face of such significantly altered neuroanatomy and neuropathology, or (f) rely on clinical interviews with informants like family or staff who are with the person regularly. These patient presentations involve so much extensive and global impairment, which is tremendously overwhelming, emotionally challenging, and really hard to know where to begin. Whilst this strikes fear into new staff (and it should), it also frees you to really think about each individual person you work with. It requires you to go back to first principles, use the scientist–practitioner approach to engage a detective, forensic interest in applying knowledge from neuroanatomy, neuropathology, neuropsychological factors, psychometric, and statistical principles to create personalised assessments. You must work from an $n=1$, single-case experimental design. These skills are in a neuropsychologist's tool box. Despite the significant, extensive, and global impairment, it is possible to gather information about the person's unique strengths. Then to determine how these can be captured and harnessed to help them make choices, engage with life, and find a quality of life in the context of such severe and complex neuro-disability. We have written this book from our perspectives as consultant clinical neuropsychologists and close to 80 years of cumulative experience with this clinical population, but recognise that the themes will be helpful to others in the wider team too. Throughout this book, we refer to people with severe brain injuries as 'patients' rather than 'clients' or 'service-users'. Whilst this has its own limitations, it reflects the language of inpatient clinical settings and alludes to the people we support rarely being able to contribute and collaborate in their assessment and neurorehabilitation.

Finally, it is worth sharing that we are often asked socially when people discover what we do and who we work with, 'isn't it depressing?' and 'what can you even do for them?'. Undoubtedly this work is at times extremely sad. You bear witness to great pain and tragedies in people's lives. You are present at the end of some people's lives. You spend a great deal of time with their very distressed families. But this is important work. Having survived the unsurvivable, they are still here. It is now imperative for us all to support these people to thrive. This means being able to join with their families to seek out what can be harnessed and how to mine for the magic moments amongst all of this tragedy. We see our work as helping, even if that is to bring certainty when the diagnosis is a prolonged disorder of consciousness, which frees the family from fears that their loved person is in some way locked in.

References

All Parliamentary Group on Acquired Brain Injury. (2018). Acquired Brain Injury and Neurorehabilitation; Time for Change. United Kingdom Acquired Brain Injury Forum. cdn.ymaws.com/ukabif.org.uk/resource/resmgr/campaigns/appg-abi_report_time-for-cha.pdf

Boss, P. (2000). Ambiguous Loss. Harvard University Press.

Cipolletta, S., Pasi, M., & Avesani, R. (2016). Vita tua, mors mea: The experience of family caregivers of patients in a vegetative state. *Journal of Health Psychology*, *21*(7), 1197–1206. https://doi.org/10.1177/1359105314550348

Jennett, B., Snoek, J., Bond, M. R., & Brooks, N. (1981). Disability after severe head injury: observations on the use of the Glasgow Outcome Scale. *Journal of Neurology, Neurosurgery, and Psychiatry*, *44*(4), 285–293. https://doi.org/10.1136/jnnp.44.4.285

Kitzinger, J., & Kitzinger, C. (2013). The 'window of opportunity' for death after severe brain injury: Family experiences. *Sociology of Health & Illness*, *35*(7), 1095–1112. https://doi.org/10.1111/1467-9566.12020

Rose, A. E., Cullen, B., Crawford, S., & Evans, J. J. (2023). A systematic review of mood and depression measures in people with severe cognitive and communication impairments following acquired brain injury. *Clinical Rehabilitation*, *37*(5), 679–700. https://doi.org/10.1177/02692155221139023

Turner-Stokes, L., Scott, H., Williams, H., & Siegert, R. (2012). The Rehabilitation Complexity Scale--extended version: Detection of patients with highly complex needs. *Disability and Rehabilitation*, *34*(9), 715–720. https://doi.org/10.3109/09638288.2011.615880

2 What's in a name?

A significant challenge in the field of complex neuro-disability surrounds the definition and use of terms. Having a shared language is vital to ensure that clinicians and researchers have clarity about who and what they are talking about. Without this, there are risks that labels, care, and treatment can be applied incorrectly, with adverse impacts on patients' outcomes and well-being. However, trying to achieve universal consistency is fraught with challenges. This chapter will discuss these challenges with regard to both definitions of severity of brain injury and different diagnostic conditions. This chapter provides an overview of the legal framework that applies when providing healthcare to patients with severe brain injury in England and Wales, plus the complexities associated with keeping up to date with an evolving legal landscape.

2.1 Definitions of severity of brain injury

'Severe' brain injury is often poorly defined. Many definitions focus solely on the initial severity of the insult of the traumatic brain injury (TBI) rather than on longer-term outcomes across a broader range of causes of acquired brain injury (ABI). Focusing initially on TBI, measures of severity of the initial injury include the Glasgow Coma Scale (GCS), duration of loss of consciousness, duration of post-traumatic amnesia (PTA), or combinations of these methods into a composite score.

The GCS provides a gross measure of awareness by examining a person's responsiveness in three domains – motor, verbal, and visual. It is a quick assessment that can be carried out at the scene of an injury, examining the extent to which a person can respond. Scores range from 3 to 15 with higher scores associated with lower injury severity; a score of 15 indicates that the person can spontaneously open their eyes, obey motor commands, and demonstrate orientation to person, place, and time. In contrast, the lowest score of 3 is obtained when the person cannot open their eyes, make sounds, or move their limbs even with prompting. Scores of 13–15 are rated as 'mild', 9-12 'moderate', and 3-8 'severe', a classification system that has remained

DOI: 10.4324/9781032665986-2

consistent since the original development in the 1970s (Teasdale & Jennett, 1974). A recent review not only concluded that the GCS remains the main tool used for classifying the severity of TBI but also highlighted that there is wide acceptance of its limitations, particularly that it cannot capture specific features of a person's brain injury and that scores are affected by non-brain injury factors such as alcohol or drug consumption and sedation or other medications (Maas et al., 2022).

Duration of loss of consciousness following the initial injury is self-explanatory. Unsurprisingly, mild TBI is defined by either no loss of consciousness or only a short duration (less than 30 minutes), whereas severe TBI is linked with hours or even days of loss of consciousness, although some classification systems differentiate between 'severe' and 'very severe'. The duration of loss of consciousness can also be affected by the treatments provided, such as sedation, anaesthetics, and other medications.

PTA is the length of time post-injury in which the person presents in a confused and disorientated state. The person is said to have emerged from PTA once they are fully orientated with continuous memory. Use of the term 'PTA' is particularly challenging when applied to people with severe to profound brain injury whose deficits in orientation and memory may endure without ever fully resolving. This issue is described in more detail later in the chapter, but for the purpose of defining the severity of the acute injury, PTA lasting less than an hour is classified as 'mild' TBI, between an hour and a day as 'moderate', and durations of longer than 24 hours as 'severe', with some classifications also considering PTA of longer than a week to denote a 'very severe' TBI. Whilst PTA is a commonly used marker of initial injury severity, it is important to note that it is not always assessed and recorded accurately at the time of the incident and can be impacted by medications, alcohol, and drugs. More commonly PTA is established retrospectively by a combination of inference from past medical records and the patient's self-report at the time of interview; it is therefore a potentially unreliable measure (Friedland & Swash, 2016; Tenovuo et al., 2021).

It has been acknowledged that none of the three measures described above may be sufficient alone to determine severity, and evidence suggests that combining information from a range of different sources provides better sensitivity and specificity. For example, the Mayo Classification System for TBI severity (Malec et al., 2007) combines available data from sources including GCS scores, PTA, duration of loss of consciousness, and neuro-imaging evidence of structural injury to arrive at an overall score for severity of a three-point scale: 'Moderate-Severe (Definite) TBI', 'Mild (Probable) TBI', and 'Symptomatic (Possible) TBI'.

More recently, there has been increased awareness that a broad spectrum of factors, including the extent of extracranial injury, metabolic and blood biomarkers, neuroimaging findings, and genetic and demographic factors, may all potentially be of use both in guiding optimal acute care for the person and in predicting longer-term outcome (Maas et al., 2022). It has been argued that even combination models have limited predictive power due to the wide range of biological, genetic, psychological, and social factors that contribute to outcome (Tenovuo et., 2021). An international working group has made a first attempt to create a single standardised methodology for combining this data into a measure of acute traumatic brain injury severity. This new CBI-M framework has recently been proposed to capture this multi-dimensional characterisation of TBI in the acute traumatic brain injury stage (Manley et al., 2025) with four pillars: a clinical pillar (full GCS and pupillary reactivity); a biomarker pillar (blood-based measures); an imaging pillar (pathoanatomical measures); and a modified pillar (features influencing clinical presentation and outcome)

The methods referred to above describe methods of classifying TBI and are not necessarily transferable to other types of acute onset brain injuries such as stroke or anoxia. UK clinical guidelines on the initial management of stroke focus on rapid diagnosis to ensure appropriate treatment is delivered as quickly as possible (NICE, 2022). To this end, initial diagnostic screening approaches such as F.A.S.T. at the scene (Face, Arm, Speech, Time; Department of Health, 2009), and ROSIER on arrival at the hospital (Recognition of Stroke in the Emergency Room; Nor et al., 2005) are used to determine the likelihood that symptoms are due to stroke, and thus enable fast access to a specialist stroke setting, appropriate imaging, and pharmacological and other treatments. This focus on the differential diagnosis of the presence/absence of stroke is important given that treatment options differ between ischaemic and haemorrhagic stroke, and the risks of mortality and longer-term disability are reduced by providing the right treatment as quickly as possible (NICE, 2022); however, these screening tools are not used as measures of severity per se.

Other measurement tools that are applied in the acute stroke setting include the GCS (described above) and the National Institutes of Health and Stroke Scale (NIHSS, Ortiz & Sacco, 2014). The NIHSS provides a classification of stroke from minor to severe based on bedside evaluation of a range of factors such as consciousness, motor ability, language, and so on; a score between 21 and 42 denotes 'severe stroke'. These measures of initial severity are used most commonly in acute settings as part of the decision-making process around the most appropriate treatments (NICE, 2022) but are not necessarily applied to outcomes in the longer term.

Regardless of the method(s) used to define initial injury severity, it remains the case that the severity at injury does not map neatly onto the severity of the outcome. In the acute stage, many medical doctors accept that occasionally patients will make a good recovery, despite poor early prognostic signs. This creates a level of uncertainty in prognostication. Thus, some seemingly relatively mild injuries in the immediate acute setting can result in significant long-term difficulties, whilst some very severe initial presentations result in apparently complete recovery (Tenovuo et al., 2021). The same authors argue that the severity of the outcome may vary depending on the viewpoint of the observer. They gave an example in which a person sustained a life-threatening initial injury but went on to regain full independence with core activities of daily living. In this scenario, their neurosurgeon might judge their ongoing deficits to be mild, whereas the neuropsychologist might judge the deficits to be severe based on neuropsychological assessment, and their family might judge their ongoing difficulties to be profound based on changes in emotions and personality (Tenovuo et al., 2021).

This challenge was highlighted in a systematic review of measures of mood and depression in people with severe brain injury (Rose et al., 2022), which showed a lack of consistency in definitions across studies, such that many participants categorised as having 'severe' brain injury presented with only moderate difficulties in the longer term – for example, having sufficient cognitive abilities to complete self-report measures over the phone or being able to complete written questionnaires independently and return them by mail. Thus, some people whose initial brain injury is classified as 'severe' will make a seemingly full functional recovery, whereas others will be left with significant physical, cognitive, and communication difficulties. Further, for those grouped by a 'severe' descriptor, this cohort of the most profoundly and catastrophically injured is not specifically captured.

2.2 Ways of measuring severity of outcome

There are other measures that attempt to capture the severity of the outcome as opposed to the severity of the acute injury. These include the Glasgow Outcome Scale (GOS), Ranchos Los Amigos Scale, Modified Rankin Scale, and some of the measures used routinely across UK rehabilitation centres. In addition, there are frameworks such as that developed by the World Health Organisation (WHO), which guide clinicians on how to separate the physical effects of an injury from its impact on the person's daily life. These approaches are outlined briefly below.

The GOS was designed as a broad overview of disability outcomes following TBI. The original version of the scale had five points on which the lowest score of 1 indicated that the patient had died, with the highest score of 5 denoting 'good recovery'. (Jennett & Bond, 1975). This scale was later extended to an eight-point scale (Glasgow Outcome Scale Extended; GOSE, Jennett et al., 1981) in order to delineate more clearly between those with different levels of moderate to severe disability (scores 3–6), and those who had made a good recovery needing no support versus those whose good recovery was within a context of variability or some reduction in activity (scores 7 and 8). Subsequent work showed evidence of poor agreement on the GOSE between clinicians from different disciplines, leading to the creation of an interview to support assessment, and then a manual containing additional advice on how to deal with 'borderline' scores (Wilson et al., 2021). The patient group we are discussing in this book would score between a GOSE score of 2 ('vegetative state') up to a maximum of 5 ('lower moderate disability'), with most scoring 3 ('lower severe disability') due to ongoing dependence on others. This narrow range of scores helps to illustrate why although this measure has a range of uses, particularly in grouping patients for the purpose of research studies, it has limited utility in helping understand the needs of individual patients.

An alternative outcome scale used in TBI is the Ranchos Los Amigos Scale (RLAS). This scale was developed as an eight-point scale to examine cognitive and behavioural difficulties rather than physical disabilities (Hagen et al., 1972), and it was later expanded to a 10-point scale (RLAS-R: Ranchos Los Amigos Revised Scale). Using Roman numerals, scores range from I ('No response/total assistance') to X ('Purposeful, appropriate/moderate independent'). The patient group we are discussing in this book would score between a I ('no response') and a IV ('confused-agitated response'). This scale can aid clinicians in having a shared language for labelling different levels of difficulty; however, similar to the GOSE, these broad labels of overall ability level have limited value when trying to understand a person's areas of strengths and weaknesses, which also limits use for planning appropriate management and intervention.

Similar ordinal scales have been developed to classify brain injuries other than TBI. For example, the widely used Modified Rankin Scale (mRS; Banks & Marotta, 2007) provides a measure of disability resulting from stroke on a scale ranging from 0 (no symptoms) to 6 (dead). This scale is reported to have significant value in stroke-related clinical trials and quality improvement projects (Saver et al., 2021) but has similar limitations to the TBI scales described above when applied to a neurorehabilitation setting. An equivalent measure in anoxic brain injuries, with similar advantages and disadvantages, is the Glasgow-Pittsburgh Cerebral Performance Category Scale (CPS), which provides a broad classification of outcome following resuscitation after a cardiac arrest on a five-point scale ranging from 1 ('good cerebral performance') to 5 ('brain dead') (Raina et al., 2008).

Thus, overall, the most commonly used outcome scales for classifying the severity of acquired brain injuries have limited utility in rehabilitation settings, which is unsurprising given that this is not the purpose for which they were designed.

Other potential measures of severity include outcome measures, which are used in rehabilitation settings. For example, in the UK, all designated post-acute Level 1 neurorehabilitation services must complete the National Dataset for Specialist Rehabilitation Services, which are collated by the UK Rehabilitation Outcomes Collaborative (UKROC). As this dataset applies to all patients within these services, regardless of aetiology, the tools were designed to be multi-purpose rather than specific to, e.g. TBI or stroke. The set includes a measure of complexity: the Extended Rehabilitation Complexity Scale (ERCS; Turner-Stokes et al., 2012), two measures of input, examining nursing needs (Northwick Park Dependency Score; Turner-Stokes et al., 1998) and therapy input (Northwick Park Therapy Dependency Assessment; Turner-Stokes et al., 2009), and an outcome measure that captures the extent to which patients return to independent functioning across a wide range of physical and cognitive domains (FIMFAM, Turner-Stokes et al., 1999).

These measures potentially have a wide range of uses in terms of allocating patients to the correct service for their needs, demonstrating the functional gains, and cost savings achieved when rehabilitation has resulted in significant gains and providing evidence to commissioners of the clinical input needed across disciplines. However, their use is more limited when applied to patients who continue to present with significant disabilities throughout their rehabilitation and beyond, such as many of those we are talking about in this book. These measures also have significant limitations when it comes to understanding the strengths, weaknesses, and interventions needed for individual patients. For example, two patients can present with the same score but very different needs. At the most extreme end, a patient in a vegetative state (VS) who remains in a VS will show no change in FIMFAM scores between admission and discharge despite having received intensive input from a specialist team. The UKROC measures are therefore useful but insufficient for clearly defining this patient group and determining which management and intervention strategies are needed for each person.

Another framework that is widely used in neurorehabilitation is the World Health Organisation's International Classification of Function (ICF; WHO, 2001). This framework illustrates that any disability resulting from a health condition is a function not just of the diagnosis and the impairments caused by its physiological impact on the body but also of how the condition and related impairments impact a person's ability to engage with activities and participate in daily life. The framework also includes consideration of the environmental and personal factors that influence impairments, activity, and participation. An example of how this framework can be applied to neuropsychological interventions was provided in a recent overview of such interventions (Wong et al., 2023). In their example, the health condition affecting the brain was an ABI, and the resulting impairment was in memory functioning. They argued that although the memory impairment could be quantified using a neuropsychological assessment, the aim of neuropsychological intervention would not be to improve the scores on a test but to improve activity and participation. In their example, the activity limitation was that the person was forgetting appointments, and the participation restrictions were that they were unable to return to work. Thus, the aim of intervention would be to teach the patient strategies for remembering appointments and support them with applying these strategies in the workplace, in order for them to be able to go back to work. A successful intervention would be measured by any return to work, regardless of any changes or otherwise on memory test scores.

This model is a useful reference point when considering whether a goal has personal meaning for the person and/or whether it will enhance their quality of life, and the importance of personalised goal setting is discussed in more detail in Chapter 3. However, it is insufficient by itself to guide which intervention strategies are likely to be of most use to the person. There is thus another step needed, which is an individualised formulation. This was illustrated in the paper referred to above by means of three hypothetical cases, all of whom presented with memory difficulties that impacted upon activity and participation but required different interventions based on factors such as their broader cognitive profile, insight into their difficulties, mood, fatigue, motivation, extent of family support, substance use, and comorbid medical conditions (Wong et al., 2023). Thus, although the measurement tools discussed in this section may be useful in many circumstances, within a neurorehabilitation setting, understanding injury severity, its impact on the person's functioning, and how best to help and support them, requires skills in psychological formulation. The importance of formulation and how to do it well is discussed throughout this book and specifically in Chapter 7.

2.3 Challenges with diagnostic labels

The purpose of a diagnostic label is to promote a shared language and understanding between clinicians, researchers, and the public as to the features of a particular condition (its signs and symptoms) and the implications of these, including the range of possible treatments and the prognosis for recovery. In order to promote this shared language, there are international diagnostic manuals such as the Diagnostic and Statistical Manual for Mental Disorders (DSM-5-TR, American Psychological Association, 2022), which focuses on mental health (including some conditions affecting neuro-cognitive functioning such as TBI) and the International Classification of Diseases for Mortality and Morbidity Statistics (ICD-11, World Health Organisation, 2018) which takes a broader approach including physical as well as mental illnesses. Chapter 8 of the ICD-11 focuses on diseases of the nervous system, including TBI, strokes, tumours, and neuro-degenerative conditions. It should be highlighted that in this cohort of patients many will no longer have typical neuroanatomy, and therefore, the applicability of these models requires caution.

There is also a wide range of specific diagnostic labels that are applied within the field of severe brain injury, and some of these conditions are considered in more detail in this book, including locked-in-syndrome and prolonged disorders of consciousness (PDOC), such as VS and minimally conscious states (MCS). It is important to note that in addition to the challenges associated with defining a 'severe' brain injury, which were outlined earlier in this chapter, there are also controversies around the use of diagnostic labels. Some challenges with these labels include different use of terminology across countries; for example, the terms 'vegetative state', 'apallic syndrome', and 'unresponsive wakefulness syndrome' are different terms for the same condition (von Wild et al., 2012). There are also inconsistencies in applications of subdivisions of diagnostic categories; for example, the subdivision of MCS into MCS+ and MCS− (Bruno et al., 2011) is applied in some studies and guidelines but not others. There are also controversies around the boundaries of whether a patient falls within a particular category or not; for an example of this, see the discussion on definitions of emergence from PDOC in Chapter 8. Another challenge within the field of neurorehabilitation is when diagnostic labels from other areas such as mental health are applied to people with ABI, with the assumption that the label carries the same implications as it does within the non-brain injured population. There is evidence that such assumptions may not be justified with people with severe brain injury; for example, a survey of over 30 clinicians with experience working with such patients found a common theme of skepticism about whether the concept of depression could be applied in the same way to people with severe brain injury to those with less severe or no brain injuries (Rose et al., 2024). For example, there is a long history of criticism of psychiatric labels such as schizophrenia, with claims that such labels lack reliability and validity (e.g. Bentall et al., 1988), and that individualised psychological formulation is a better alternative (e.g. Johnstone, 2017). Criticisms also include evidence that diagnostic labels can be associated with stigma and stereotypes, and there is some evidence that fears of stigma extend to those with neurological conditions and can impact negatively on participation in daily life (e.g. Hagger & Riley, 2019; Bracho Ponce & Salas, 2024).

From a clinical perspective, we have also observed instances where labels associated with disorders of motivation and initiation such as 'akinetic mutism' or 'abulia' have been incorrectly applied to people in PDOC, potentially affecting both treatment planning and the expectations of both clinicians and families. Similar challenges are noted when the label of 'locked in syndrome' has been applied to patients with severe global cognitive impairment, in spite of intact cognition being a key criterion in the definition of the syndrome; this is discussed in more detail in Chapter 9. Similarly, we have encountered particular challenges around the use of the label PTA. As discussed earlier in this chapter, PTA is defined as the duration of confusion and disorientation following a TBI, with emergence from PTA determined by the return of orientation and continuous memory. However, this definition assumes that resolution will occur, whereas, for this cohort of patients, this may not ever be the case. Challenges with the label of PTA have been recognized elsewhere, including proposals to use the term 'post traumatic confusional state' (PTCS) rather than PTA given that symptoms extend beyond amnesia (Sherer et al., 2020). These authors acknowledged that for some patients in PTCS, their cognitive impairments may never recover but argued that there is currently no clear consensus on how to label this phenomenon nor on when to determine that the enduring nature of their difficulties means that the label of PTCS (or PTA) no longer applies. The challenge around these uncertainties in a neurorehabilitaton setting is that clinicians may continue assessing for PTA – i.e. repeatedly asking questions related to orientation and memory – when there is no longer any realistic prospect of the patient spontaneously recovering these abilities. For such patients, rehabilitation strategies focusing on compensating for their memory deficits and/or teaching them key pieces of information via strategies such as error-less learning may be more appropriate.

Overall, diagnostic labels remain an essential means of shared language both between clinicians and between clinicians and families, but caution is needed in applying them correctly and in ensuring that an open-minded approach is taken to understanding each patient's individual presentation, without basing expectations too rigidly around their diagnosis.

2.4 Providing clinical care within an evolving legal landscape

When providing care and treatment to people with severe brain injuries, there are two major pieces of legislation to be aware of within England and Wales, namely the Mental Health Act (MHA, 1983; amended 2007) and the Mental Capacity Act (MCA, 2005). Both of these pieces of legislation provide legal frameworks for treating people without their explicit consent, along-side the safeguards needed to ensure that this is only done in circumstances in which it is judged absolutely necessary. An in-depth knowledge of the MCA is necessary (see the British Psychological Society (BPS), 2019) when working with patients with severe brain injury, as described below. However, it is important for clinicians to also be aware of the MHA and the bound-aries between the two acts. The MHA is concerned with diagnosable mental health disorders (e.g. schizophrenia, bipolar disorder, severe depression), and the actions needed to provide emergency or urgent treatment if the disorder leads the person to behave in a way that causes immediate risk of significant harm to themselves or others. In contrast, the MCA provides a framework for how to act in someone's best interests when they are assessed as lacking the mental capacity to make that decision for themselves. It follows that there are situations in which someone with a mental health disorder may also lack the capacity to make decisions and/or that someone who presents as lacking the capacity to make a decision about their treatment may also be determined to have an underlying mental health disorder, i.e. there is overlap between the two acts. The MCA provides specific guidance in Section 28 about this interface, which clarifies that if a person is detained under the MHA then it is the MHA rather than the MCA, which applies. In circumstances in which the person is not already detained and there is debate about which legislation is most appropriate, then careful consideration is needed; the MCA Code of Practice (2007; Chapter 13) provides detailed guidance on this.

In order to understand how the MCA is applied when working with patients with severe brain injury, the first point to consider is that in most clinical settings, including those treating people with mild to moderate brain injury, care and treatment are provided within a framework of informed consent. Clinicians provide their patients with information about diagnosis and prognosis, explain what care and treatment is on offer, what they are recommending and why, and seek explicit informed consent for the treatment plan from the intended recipient. However, not all patients are able to provide informed consent for one or more aspects of their treatment plan, and the MCA exists to safe-guard such people. Elsewhere in the United Kingdom, equivalent principles of mental capacity are outlined in The Adults with Incapacity (Scotland) Act (2000) and The Mental Capacity Act (Northern Ireland) (2016). Whilst there are some differences in legislation between the devolved UK nations, the key principles are broadly consistent. Thus, a person's mental capacity to make decisions for themselves should generally be presumed unless there is clear reason to question this. However, when there is reason for concern, i.e. there is clear evidence of a 'disorder of mind or brain', which is impacting upon the person's ability to make decisions (which will be the case for the vast majority of people with severe brain injury), then an assessment of mental capacity must be undertaken. Clinicians undertaking such assessments must be clear about the specific decision in question and the information that is pertinent to that decision in order to carry out a decision-specific functional test of cap-acity. This entails assessing the patient's ability to understand, retain, and use and weigh the information pertinent to the decision, in order to then commu-nicate a clear decision. Decisions relevant to this patient group might include consenting to an inpatient admission to a neurorehabilitation service, making day-to-day treatment or care decisions such as taking their medication or receiving personal care, or more complex decisions such as making informed choices about discharge planning or life-sustaining treatments.

Other key principles of the legislation and associated codes of practice are that people should be given support to make their own decisions, for example, adapting assessment techniques (e.g. using pictorial or written aids, repetition of information, choosing the optimal environment and time of day for the person), and that people have the right to make decisions that others might consider 'unwise'. It is therefore extremely important to have a robust formulation of the person's cognitive and communicative strengths and weaknesses and any strategies that optimise their strengths, particularly when attempting to determine whether a person lacks capacity versus making an 'unwise' but capacitous decision. The MCA Code of Practice (2007) provides practical guidance on some of these strategies, whilst also outlining when specialist input from professionals such as speech and language therapists or clinical neuropsychologists may be warranted (MCA Code of Practice section 3.11). Whilst professionals may frequently carry out such assessments indi-vidually, within an inpatient setting, complex mental capacity assessments may be undertaken jointly. For example, an SLT and clinical psychologist may work together to assess a patient who presents with a combination of communication, memory, and executive difficulties due to the SLT's experi-ence in supporting communication deficits and the psychologist's expertise in learning, memory, and executive functioning. Joint working with other professionals within the team may also be indicated, e.g. occupational therapists may provide observations around patients' behaviour in functional tasks, which may help determine if there is a dissociation between what the patient says they will do and what they actually do in practice (a 'knowing/

doing' dissociation, also referred to as the 'frontal lobe paradox'; George & Gilbert, 2018). Nevertheless, even with optimal specialist support, people with severe and/or profound brain injury are likely to lack the capacity to make some, most, or even all decisions for themselves.

When people lack the capacity to make their own decisions, the MCA (2005) outlines how to act in the person's best interests, in a way that is least restrictive of their rights and freedoms. Some key best interests decisions for this patient group are described briefly below, although it is important to note that best interests decision-making does not apply to all types of scenarios. For example, the MCA does not permit anyone to make decisions around sexual activity and marriage on behalf of another person. In addition, there are scenarios in which decisions relating to clinical care and treatment are not subject to best interests decision-making. These include those for which the incapacitated person made a valid and applicable advance decision prior to their brain injury, such as an advance decision to refuse treatment (ADRT), and situations in which one or more people hold decision-making power, either through being appointed by the person before they lost capacity (e.g. a Lasting Power of Attorney (LPA)) or by the courts (e.g. a court-appointed deputy (CAD)). In these scenarios, there is an obligation for the treating clinical team to check the legitimacy and applicability of the appointment and, where third parties are involved, to ensure that they are given the relevant information needed to make decisions on the person's behalf, but the clinicians are not able to override them; in the rare event of there being serious concerns that an LPA or CAD is planning a course of action that appears to be against the patient's best interests, then advice should be sought from the court.

In our clinical experience, we have encountered only a small number of patients who had set up an advance decision or LPA prior to their injury. More commonly, as clinical neuropsychologists with specialist skills in understanding cognitive functioning, we might carry out assessments of mental capacity in relation to a patient's ability to choose one or people to act as their LPA subsequent to their brain injury (whether this is for health and welfare decisions, financial decisions, or both), and if the patient lacks capacity, we might be asked to complete paperwork to confirm this (a COP3 form), which will be submitted to the Court of the Protection as part of an application to enable a CAD to be appointed to act on the person's behalf. Unless and until a valid LPA or CAD is in place, all aspects of care and treatment for which the person lacks capacity will be subject to best interests decision-making.

Best interests decisions are usually made by the most senior health or social care professional responsible for enacting the decision in consultation with the person's family and friends, any independent mental capacity advocates, and the broader clinical team. These decisions must also involve consideration of any current preferences the person themselves can express and a wider consideration of their wishes, preferences, beliefs, and values, placing these at the heart of the decision-making process where possible. Two particular types of best interests decisions are outlined in more detail below; the first of these outlines the applicability of deprivation of liberty safeguards (DoLs) to this patient group, while the second concerns the ethically sensitive area of best interests decision-making in relation to life-sustaining treatments.

When the best interests decision is around an admission for inpatient care and treatment, including for rehabilitation, then the clinical team must determine whether any restrictions are being placed upon the person's liberty, which might include both physical and chemical constraints. Physical constraints might include raising cotsides on a hospital bed, tray tables, headbands to keep the person's head upright in a wheelchair, tilt-in-space wheelchairs, abdominal binders to prevent PEG tube removal, or mittens to prevent scratching/ dislodging of tubes. Chemical restraints might include medications prescribed for the purpose of reducing behaviours such as physical aggression or serious self-harm. Since the Cheshire West ruling (P v Cheshire West & Chester Council & Another, 2014), a deprivation of liberty is also considered to occur whenever someone who cannot provide informed consent and is under 24-hour supervision would be prevented from leaving if they attempted to do so. This applies whether or not the person has made active attempts to leave and whether or not they are physically capable of doing so, and therefore applies to many people with severe brain injury, including those in PDOC. Under UK law, Deprivation of Liberty Safeguards (DoLs) are required to be put in place to protect vulnerable people by ensuring that any restrictions on their liberty are necessary and proportionate in their best interests.

Best interests decision-making in relation to life-sustaining treatments can apply to a range of treatments, including whether to place someone on a ventilator to support breathing or whether to prescribe antibiotics to treat a severe infection. More controversially, it also applies to the delivery of clinically assisted nutrition and hydration (CANH). CANH is classed in UK law as a medical treatment rather than as 'food and water' and, as such, it is subject to consideration under the MCA when the person receiving it cannot give informed consent to receive it. Both clinicians and families can find this definition conceptually and ethically challenging, and discussions around whether ongoing CANH is in the person's best interests require considerable skill to navigate, particularly given that death is the inevitable outcome should treatment be discontinued. In the relatively recent past in the UK, CANH was only discontinued in cases with a confirmed diagnosis of 'permanent vegetative state' after a court hearing (see MCA Code of Practice sections 6.18, 8.18, and 8.19). However, more recent case law shifted the emphasis away from specific diagnostic labels towards a broader understanding of best interests in terms of a quality of life that the person themselves would value (Aintree v James; Briggs v Briggs). In addition, it has since been established that when there is consensus that ongoing treatment would not be in the person's best interests (such as withholding or discontinuing CANH from a person in PDOC), a court hearing is not required provided that rigorous professional practice guidance is followed (Supreme Court ~ A NHS Trust v Y

[2018] UKSC 46). When there is disagreement about best interests in relation to CANH, or the decision is finely balanced, an application to court is still required (BMA, 2018). The third potential scenario is that there is consensus that ongoing treatment remains in the individual person's best interests; in this case, treatment will obviously continue, although case law has clarified the need for continual monitoring such that best interests can be reviewed if the balance of benefits and harms of treatment changes (North West London CCG v GU).

Detailed professional practice guidelines are invaluable in understanding the legal processes and application of the MCA in relation to ongoing CANH, and these specify three groups of patients to which these apply: (1) patients in PDOC following a sudden onset brain injury (BMA 2018, RCP 2020), (2) patients with advanced and progressing neurodegenerative disorders, and (3) those with ABI in the context of multiple co-morbidities and reduced life expectancy, who lack the capacity to make their own decisions about CANH (BMA, 2018). Nevertheless, applying these principles in real-world clinical practice requires a highly skilled team, that can support patients' families and friends through often challenging conversations around diagnosis, prognosis, and what would constitute a meaningful quality of life for a person with little or no ability to advocate for themselves, within a context where some uncertainty about these issues is inevitable. Guidance to assist clinicians with this is provided by the British Psychological Society (BPS, 2021). Additional challenges for clinicians include how to ensure that all family members are given the opportunity to communicate openly and honestly about the patient's wishes, beliefs, and values – which may not be possible within a 'best interests meeting' but may require 1:1 conversations, telephone calls, and/or written contact – and how to be as objective as possible in approach, given that all professionals will have their own personal views on such ethically complex issues (Olgiati et al., 2023). These issues are discussed further in Chapter 8.

References

American Psychiatric Association. (2022). Diagnostic and Statistical Manual of Mental Disorders (5th ed., text rev.). https://doi.org/10.1176/appi.books.9780890425787

Banks, J. L., & Marotta, C. A. (2007). Outcomes validity and reliability of the modified Rankin scale: Implications for stroke clinical trials: a literature review and synthesis. *Stroke*, 38(3), 1091–1096. https://doi.org/10.1161/01.STR.0000258355.23810.c6

Bentall, R., Jackson, H. F., & Pilgrim, D. (1988). Abandoning the concept of 'schizophrenia': Some implications of validity arguments for psychological research into psychotic phenomena. *British Journal of Clinical Psychology*, 27 (4), 303–324. https://doi.org/10.1111/j.2044-8260.1988.tb00795.x

BMA/RCP. (2018). Clinically-assisted nutrition and hydration (CANH) and adults who lack the capacity to consent: Guidance for decision-making in England and Wales. www.bma.org.uk/media/1161/bma-clinically-assisted-nutrition-hydration-canh-full-guidance.pdf

Bracho Ponce, M. J., & Salas, C. (2024). The many faces of stigma after acquired brain injury: A systematic review. *Brain Impairment, 25*. https://doi.org/10.1071/IB23076

British Psychological Society (BPS). (2019). *What Makes a Good Assessment of Mental Capacity?*. Mental Capacity Advisory Group, BPS. https://doi.org/10.53841/bps rep.2019.rep127

British Psychological Society (BPS). (2021). *Supporting People who Lack Mental Capacity: A guide to Best Interest's Decision Making.* Mental Capacity Advisory Group, BPS. https://doi.org/10.53841/bpsrep.2022.inf149

Bruno, M. A, Vanhaudenhuyse, A., Thibaut, A., Moonen, G., & Laureys, S. (2011). From unresponsive wakefulness to minimally conscious PLUS and functional locked-in syndromes: Recent advances in our understanding of disorders of consciousness. *Journal of Neurology, 258*(7), 1373–1384. https://doi.org/10.1007/s00 415-011-6114-x

Department of Health. (1987). Mental Health Act. London: HM SO.

Department of Health. (2005). Mental Capacity Act. London: HMSO.

Department of Health. (2009). Stroke: Act F.A.S.T. awareness campaign. Available at: http://webarchive.nationalarchives.gov.uk/20130107105354/http://www.dh.gov.uk/en/Publicationsandstatistics/Publications/PublicationsPolicyAndGuidance/DH_094239

Friedland, D., & Swash, M, (2016). Post-traumatic amnesia and confusional state: Hazards of retrospective assessment. *Journal of Neurology, Neurosurgery and Psychiatry, 87*, 1068–1074.

George, M., & Gilbert, S. (2018). Mental Capacity Act (2005) assessments. Why everyone needs to know about the frontal lobe paradox. *The Neuropsychologist, 5*, 59–66.

Hagen, C., Malkmus, D., & Durham, P. (1972). *Levels of cognitive functioning.* Rancho Los Amigos Hospital.

Hagger, B. F., & Riley, G. A. (2019). The social consequences of stigma-related self-concealment after acquired brain injury. *Neuropsychological Rehabilitation, 29*(7), 1129–1148. https://doi.org/10.1080/09602011.2017.1375416

Jennett, B., and & Bond, M. (1975). Assessment of outcome after severe brain damage. A practical scale. *Lancet, 305*, 480–484.

Jennett, B., Snoek, J., Bond, M. R., and & Brooks, N. (1981). Disability after severe head injury: Observations on the use of the Glasgow Outcome Scale. *Journal of Neurology, Neurosurgery and Psychiatry, 44*, 285–293.

Johnstone, L. (2017). Psychological formulation as an alternative to psychiatric diagnosis. *Journal of Humanistic Psychology, 58* (1). 30–46. https://doi.org/10.1177/0022167817722230

Maas, A. I. R., Menon, D. K., Manley, G. T., Abrams, M., Åkerlund, C., Andelic, N., et al., (2022). Traumatic brain injury: Progress and challenges in prevention, clinical care, and research. *The Lancet Neurology, 21*(11), 1004–1060. https://doi.org/10.1016/S1474-4422(22)00309-X

Malec, J. F., Brown, A. W., Leibson, C. L., Flaada, J. T., Mandrekar, J. N., Diehl, N. N., & Perkins, P. K. (2007). The Mayo classification system for traumatic brain injury severity. *Journal of Neurotrauma, 24*(9), 1417–1424. https://doi.org/10.1089/neu.2006.0245

Manley, G. T., Dams-O'Connor, K., Alosco, M. L., Awwad, H. O., Bazarian, J. J., Bragge, P., Corrigan, J. D., Doperalski, A., Ferguson, A. R., Mac Donald, C. L., Menon, D. K., McNett, M. M., van der Naalt, J., Nelson, L. D., Pisică, D., Silverberg, N. D.,

Umoh, N., Wilson, L., Yuh, E. L., Zetterberg, H., ... NIH-NINDS TBI Classification and Nomenclature Initiative (2025). A new characterisation of acute traumatic brain injury: The NIH-NINDS TBI Classification and Nomenclature Initiative. *The Lancet. Neurology, 24*(6), 512–523. https://doi.org/10.1016/S1474-4422(25)00154-1

NICE. (2022). NICE guideline [NG128] Stroke and transient ischaemic attack in over 16s: diagnosis and initial management.

Nor, A. M., Davis, J., Sen, B., Shipsey, D., Louw, S. J., Dyker, A.G., Davis, M., & Ford, G. A. (2005). The Recognition of Stroke in the Emergency Room (ROSIER) scale: Development and validation of a stroke recognition instrument. *Lancet Neurology, 4*, 727–734.

Office of the Public Guardian. (2007). Mental Capacity Act Code of Practice. https://assets.publishing.service.gov.uk/media/5f6cc6138fa8f541f6763295/Mental-capacity-act-code-of-practice.pdf.

Olgiati, E., Hinchliffe, J., Hanrahan, A., Mantovani, P., & Crawford, S. (2023). Ethical and practical issues for the psychologist working with patients in a disorder of consciousness. In: Fish, J., Betteridge, S., and & Wilson, B. A. (Eds). *Rare Conditions, Diagnostic Challenges and Controversies in Clinical Neuropsychology*. Routledge.

Ortiz, G.A. & Sacco, R. L. (2014). National Institutes of Health Stroke Scale (NIHSS). Wiley Online Library. https://doi.org/10.1002/9781118445112.stat06823

Raina, K. D., Callaway, C., Rittenberger, J. C., & Holm, M. B (2008). Neurological and functional status following cardiac arrest: Method and tool utility. *Resuscitation, 79*(2), 249–256. https://doi.org/10.1016/j.resuscitation.2008.06.005

Rose, A. E., Cullen, B., Crawford, S., & Evans, J. J. (2022). A systematic review of mood and depression measures in people with severe cognitive and communication impairments following acquired brain injury. *Clinical Rehabilitation, 37*(5), 679–700. https://doi.org/10.1177/02692155221139023

Rose, A. E., Cullen, B., Crawford, S., & Evans, J. J. (2024). Assessment of mood after severe acquired brain injury: Interviews with UK clinical psychologists and medical professionals. *Clinical Rehabilitation, 38*(11), 1521–1533. https://doi.org10.1177/02692155241278289

Royal College of Physicians (RCP). (2020). *Prolonged disorders of consciousness following sudden onset brain injury: National clinical guidelines*. RCP. www.rcp.ac.uk/media/ptcoggi5/pdoc-guidelines_final_online_0_0.pdf

Saver, J. L., Chaisinanunkul, N., Campbell, B. C. V., Grotta, J. C., Hill, M. D., Khatri, P., Landen, J., Lansberg, M. G., Venkatasubramanian, C., Albers, G. W., & XIth Stroke Treatment Academic Industry Roundtable (2021). Standardized nomenclature for modified Rankin Scale Global Disability outcomes: Consensus recommendations from stroke therapy academic industry roundtable XI. *Stroke, 52*(9), 3054–3062. https://doi.org/10.1161/STROKEAHA.121.034480

Sherer, M., Katz, D. I., Bodien, Y. G., Arciniegas, D. B., Block, C., Blum, S., et al,. (2020). Post-traumatic Confusional State: A case definition and diagnostic criteria. *Archives of Physical Medicine and Rehabilitation, 101*, 2041–2050. https://Doi.org/10.1016/j.apmr.2020.06.021

Teasdale, G., & Jennett, B. (1974). Assessment of coma and impaired consciousness. A practical scale. *Lancet, 2*, 81–84.

Tenovuo, O., Diaz-Arrastia, R., Goldstein, L. E., Sharp, D. J., van der Naalt, J., Zasler, N. D. (2021). Assessing the severity of traumatic brain injury-time for a change? *Journal of Clinical Medicine, 10*(1), 148. https://doi.org/10.3390/jcm10010148

Turner-Stokes, L., Nyein, K., Turner-Stokes, T., & Gatehouse, C. (1999). The UK FIM+ FAM: development and evaluation. Functional assessment measure. *Clinical Rehabilitation*, *13*(4), 277–287. https://doi.org/10.1191/026921599676896799

Turner-Stokes, L., Scott, H., Williams, H., & Siegert, R. (2012). The Rehabilitation Complexity Scale--extended version: Detection of patients with highly complex needs. *Disability Rehabilitation*, *34*(9), 715–720. https://doi.org/10.3109/09638 288.2011.615880

Turner-Stokes, L., Shaw, A., Law, J., & Rose, H. (2009). Development and initial validation of the Northwick Park Therapy Dependency Assessment. *Clinical Rehabilitation*, *23*(10), 922–937. https://doi.org/10.1177/0269215509337447

Turner-Stokes, L., Tonge, P., Nyein, K., Hunter M., Nielson, S., & Robinson, I. (1998). The Northwick Park Dependency Score (NPDS): A measure of nursing dependency in rehabilitation. *Clinical Rehabilitation*, *12*(4), 304–318. https://doi.org/10.1191/ 026921598669173600

von Wild, K., Laureys, S.T., Gerstenbrand, F., Dolce, G., & Onose, G. (2012). The vegetative state-a syndrome in search of a name. *Journal of Medicine and Life*, *5*(1), 3–15.

Wilson, L., Boase, K., Nelson, L. D, Temkin, N.R., Giacino, J. T., Markowitz, A. J., Maas, A., Menon, D. K., Teasdale, G., & Manley, G. T. (2021). A manual for the Glasgow Outcome Scale-extended Interview. *Journal of Neurotrauma*, *38*(17), 2435–2446. https://doi.org/10.1089/neu.2020.7527

Wong, D., Pike, K., Stolwyk, R., Allott, K., Ponsford, J., McKay, A., Longley, W., Bosboom, P., Hodge, A., Kinsella, G., & Mowszowski, L. (2023). Delivery of neuropsychological interventions for adult and older adult clinical populations: An Australian Expert Working Group Clinical Guidance Paper. *Neuropsychological Review*, *34*(4), 985–1047. https://doi.org/10.1007/s11065-023-09624-0

World Health Organisation. (2001). The International Classification of Functioning, Disability and Health (ICF). WHO.

World Health Organisation. (2018). International Classification of Diseases for Mortality and Morbidity Statistics. 11th revision. WHO.

Case law

Aintree University Hospitals NHS Foundation Trust v James – [2013] UKSC 67

Briggs v Briggs – [2016] EWCOP 53

P v Cheshire West & Chester Council and Another [2014]

An NHS Trust v Y – [2018] UKSC 46

North West London Clinical Commissioning Group v GU – [2021] EWCOP 59

3 Approaches to assessment and neurorehabilitation in complex neuro-disability

So far we have established that this book is considering the most impaired survivors of severe and profound brain injury. The terminology usually encountered when describing the outcome of brain injury does not specifically differentiate this most severely impacted group. They present with global impairments that impact all areas of functioning. Whilst there are inevitable difficulties with any attempts at categorisation, we have selected, although imperfect, to use the descriptor 'complex neuro-disability' because this sets out the great complexity, it confirms that there is neurological injury, and it implies that disabilities are likely to be lifelong. In the context of such severe global impairment, it can be difficult for clinicians whose brain injury experience is with people who present with particular deficits in the context of otherwise relatively 'normal' neurology, to conceptualise helpful assessment and rehabilitation approaches. It is very demoralising and deskilling to find that the tools that one has honed throughout a career are not useful with this group of patients. Approaching this work requires a paradigm shift. In the face of so much impairment, the aims become to find a person's abilities within the disabilities.

3.1 Clinical considerations in the design of assessments for people with complex neuro-disability

Broadly speaking, a neuropsychological assessment is used to determine the impact of a known brain-related condition on cognition, behaviour, and mood. As such, a good neuropsychological assessment will explore all these areas and is not simply a series of cognitive tests. Whilst in most settings, cognitive tests are usually central to a neuropsychological assessment to explore cognition, in complex neuro-disability, the brain injury is so severe that the tests that neuropsychologists usually reach for are completely inappropriate. Clearly, people with such catastrophic brain injury may not even have similar neuroanatomy to the test sample, which is presumed to represent the whole population, nor are most standardised psychometric assessments developed for this cohort so there is no normative comparative

DOI: 10.4324/9781032665986-3

information. It is common that people with complex neuro-disability will be unable to participate in these routine and common assessments, administration of the test stimulus materials/part of the test or finding that they perform at the floor on neuropsychological tests or batteries, all of which limit and confuse interpretation.

At this profound level of impairment, the deficits are so obvious, and it appears that it is often assumed that cognition is so globally impaired that it is not possible or not helpful to explore it at all. Behavioural observations may be made, but that too is complicated, as these patients are often extremely physically disabled, and behaviours may be sparse, hard to interpret, or be sure if behaviours are repeated. Assessing mood in complex neuro-disability is also fraught with difficulty as discussed in Chapter 6. In the light of these challenges, it is not uncommon to see cognitive functioning in reports and notes associated with people with complex neuro-disability described as having 'Severe Global Impairment' but with no further detail or see that many practitioners just determine the person is 'Not Assessable'.

In the context of Prolonged Disorders of Consciousness (PDOC), we do have assessment tools to enable and support diagnoses which can support the determination of whether a person has emerged from PDOC. Once a person is able to engage with pen and paper or computer assessments, we do have cognitive assessments that are designed to assess cognitive functioning. However, there is a group of people in between these levels who have emerged from PDOC but who remain severely disabled in one or more motor, sensory, cognitive, communicative, or functional domains and whose level of disability precludes them from the formal assessments that we might usually reach for.

This complex presentation means we are grappling with difficult challenges such as

- How can you assess someone after a traumatic brain injury who does not have intact receptive language ability?
- How can you formulate someone's abilities when they score on the floor on all the tests you give?
- How can you create a balanced neuropsychological assessment with someone who has a profound physical disability?
- How can you develop a neuropsychological assessment plan for someone who only concentrates and attends for a few minutes at a time?
- When a person fatigues fast, how do we know when their responses are no longer reliable? Is there a tipping point?
- What happens if someone goes to sleep in the middle of an assessment? Do we need to start again next time or jump in halfway through?
- If a person's responses are variable, how can we tell whether they are better than chance?
- If there is disagreement between staff or between staff and family about a person's capabilities, what should we do?

- How can one explore whether a person's presentation is dysexecutive or depressed if they are very physically impaired and have very limited communicative ability?
- Trying to get a person to eye point to indicate a decision may seem an obvious solution, unless the person has a visual impairment, but how do you know that a lack of response is a consequence of a sensory impairment or a cognitive impairment? This may seem like stating the obvious, but it is perhaps not the simple problem that it may seem at first.

We hope that the following chapters will help you to answer some of these questions. The challenge of how to assess people with complex neuro-disability is obvious, so perhaps it is more important to first consider, why assess this group at all?

3.2 Why assess at all?

In general, reasons for assessment are usually to consider one or more of the following:

1. To determine the presence, nature, and severity of cognitive dysfunction
2. To see how any difficulties differ from a person's presumed skills pre-injury
3. To see how a person performs compared to other people in their age group
4. To build a profile of strengths and weaknesses
5. To then consider how these strengths and weaknesses may affect the person's everyday life
6. To help both the person themselves and the people around them to understand their difficulties and the impact on daily life
7. To use this information to help plan treatment and rehabilitation aims
8. To use this information to modify methods to optimise and personalise the neurorehabilitation approach
9. For diagnostic information
10. To establish a baseline
11. To monitor change (improvement or deterioration) over time
12. To ensure that a person's legal right to make their own decisions about their own life is enabled
13. To ensure that a person is enabled to make their own choices in spite of any apparent disability

Whilst items 1–3 of this list may be less relevant, many of these matters still hold true in complex neuro-disability and perhaps are more critical. For example, if a very disabled and non-verbal person missing part of their skull and breathing through a tracheostomy is in front of most people, assumptions are made about their abilities to make any choices about their own life. Or, consider the case of a person who appears to be in VS with all decision-making about their life being made in their best interests including where they live and CANH continuation, but actually the person has LIS and likely to have the legal right to make all their own decisions. Thus decisions should not be made on the basis of assumptions, and assessments are needed, even when this is difficult.

Standardised tests are one tool to approach this. By using standardised materials and administration, it is possible to make inferences about neuro-psychological processes from the results obtained. It is also possible to make inferences about underlying neuropsychological processes by using structured behavioural-based examinations. Clearly, the same principles involved in standardised cognitive assessments hold true in structured behavioural-based assessment of reliability, validity, and replicability. However, in the context of such profound and complex neuro-disability, all such assessments depend on idiosyncratic, often very subtle responses, and the neuropsychologist must create a personalised and bespoke examination. As soon as an examiner creates a bespoke examination, it is critical that there are checks and balances to ensure the robustness of any tentative conclusions that can be drawn. Unfortunately, this is often not fully addressed in assessments.

3.3 What can they do?

We have seen reports that detail a list of cognitive deficits that are inferred from the behaviour or absence of behaviour of a person on a range of functional tasks, but without contextualising these observations within the global nature of the cognitive impairment. For example, only identifying sequencing problems in transfers in the context of gross executive functioning, attention, and motor deficits. This is a problematic approach because listing deficits belies the totality of the global impairments and can lead to erroneous assumptions that other functions remain intact. Using a deficit model when there is such widespread cognitive disability is unhelpful because it does not account for the extensive interaction between cognitive domains and encourages the idea that they are mutually exclusive.

Complex neuro-disability requires a paradigm shift in what we are trying to achieve through a neuropsychological assessment. In our assessments of people who have sustained this level of brain damage, we are not looking to identify deficits in cognitive functioning relative to life before their injury, or to compare the person to others of a similar age in the test population. Their deficits are obvious. Rather we are looking to identify what they _are able to do_. In other words, we are seeking to find the abilities within their disabilities. Interestingly, this aligns clinicians with many people's family members, who too are searching for evidence of things the person can still do, such as blink or move a finger or turn their head or make a sound that suggests recognition of them and the continuation of the bond between them.

Beaumont (2008) described this approach of searching for the person's skills in terms of a model in which one assumes none or only very limited cognitive functioning, but in which 'islets' of retained cognitive function are present. Beaumont (2008) posits the role of the neuropsychologist to chart these islets and attempt to extend their size and form bridges among them. For example, if a person is only able to move their finger, how can this be harnessed to help in their life? Perhaps the person could learn to operate a switch? If so, can they link cause and effect? If so, might they be able to use a switch for a call bell or to turn on music or their own television or similar? Can the switch then be used to form a basis for choice-making for questions put to them?

Once any behaviour has been observed, this forms the starting point for more detailed assessment. Given that the behaviours that we might want to try to harness may be very subtle, it's usually not easy to see them. This requires a great deal of time spent in quiet observation and time spent in observation of the person in different settings. When you see a behaviour occurring, this is often a good place to focus further observations and see if other behaviours emerge, as it is likely that behaviours are present when the person's arousal and alertness levels are higher. Once observed, the task is to work out whether or not behaviours are or might become consistent. This requires careful observation and controlling of settings and analysis. In other words, it is imperative to complete an assessment, but the nature and direction of the assessment are likely to be quite different and start at a different place.

As with all behavioural analysis, an aim will be to try to understand the purpose of any behaviour but in these circumstances, we may also be assessing whether there is any possibility of harnessing that behaviour and giving it a purpose or expanding upon a purpose that we hypothesise that it may have. Ultimately it may simply be a behaviour that we see and that is assumed to have some positive impact and that we therefore want to provide the environment that enables it to occur. This is obviously appealing in that any intervention that we apply should ultimately contribute to an improvement in quality of life, and this similarly is positive as there is more likely to be buy-in from family and staff working with the person.

It is also important to consider the reciprocity of behaviour for family members. Where they want to be involved, they generally will choose to do something with their relative that either they enjoy or that they perceive to be enjoyable or comforting for their loved one, even if the person themselves is unaware of it. For example, activities such as styling hair are usually preferred by family members to activities such as cleaning teeth. It is helpful to consider whether in these circumstances there is greater evidence of patient alertness or engagement. These activities are typically spontaneously generated by the family and can be valuable in maintaining bonds between family and the person, provided activities are not likely to be aversive to the patient.

3.3.1 Finding islets

For someone with profound brain injuries, it is even more essential to consider the impact of motor, sensory, communication, and cognitive disability when we try to establish what the islets of ability might be and how we can evaluate or monitor them. This demands creativity but also a clear understanding of the need for reproducibility. In this instance, we are trying to create a standardisation of the method as outlined in Chapter 4. We need to know what a person can do and whether they can do this consistently, and to establish that we must also know about their motor and sensory function, and how this can be used, or where it presents barriers.

In other words, when trying to work out what these islets might be and how we might use them, we are also exploring how to best understand potential barriers if we do not know whether, for example, a person is not responding because they do not understand, have not heard, cannot see, cannot move, or some combination of any or all of these factors is responsible for the lack of action. If we want to know about a person's cognitive ability, we also need to consider their arousal and alertness and the impact of fatigue and their motor and sensory abilities. How can a person indicate any response, or how can we detect a response? What does that response mean and is it reproducible and recognisable? Working these matters out highlights the need for teamwork with the sharing of assessments between all team members enabling much more helpful routes to and the ability to draw integrated conclusions about a person's abilities, responses, and engagement. Ensuring effective teamworking is discussed in Chapter 11.

3.4 Medical factors

It is given that in an ideal world a neuropsychological assessment is best completed after optimal management of comorbidities has been achieved, when the person is optimised to do their best. Common comorbidities in this population are likely to include epilepsy, diabetes, vestibular dysfunction, sunken flap syndrome, hyperreflexia, paroxysmal autonomic instability with dystonia (PAID) syndrome, and/or infections. However, this is not always possible, and it is important to consider medical factors that may impact our assessment and whether it is possible to address them and/or delay the assessment until their impact is lessened or resolved.

The matters that we might consider, over and above matters such as the treatment of infections with antibiotics and similar might be the neurosurgical skull replacement of a bone flap, treatment such as botox and tendon releases and management of medications that may have a knock-on effect on cognitive functioning such as drugs with a sedative effect like Baclofen or the use of an antipsychotic for agitation.

The impact of pain is also of great importance to consider. This might include both orthopaedic and neuropathic pain. In addition to the impact of the pain itself, there is the impact of pain medications, both positive and negative. Consider the following:

• The positive effect of pain medication on the ability to engage in any assessment.

- The timing of the session or the medication administration to gain the most benefit from this.
- The impact on cognitive functioning of some pain medications. For example, medications with sedative effects.
- The importance of positioning to manage pain.
- The impact pain can have on motoric ability where a motor response is sought.
- The use of pain stimuli to promote arousal such as stimulation of the nail bed.
- The prophylactic administration of pain medication prior to rehabilitation tasks like standing frames.

3.5 Arousal levels

With patients who may only be awake for short periods or whose fatigue levels result in very limited engagement before fatigue overwhelms them, it is important to plan carefully what one is trying to assess and how one might build flexibility into any assessment. Holding fast to a tight protocol with this clinical population cannot be assumed to result in a controlled test but may rather be a measure of a person's resilience (or otherwise) to fatigue. These assessments need to be flexible, and we need to be on our toes to be aware of not just levels of arousal but also rates of change. That way we have a chance to explore the most important matters before the person we are assessing needs to stop. Arousal levels are affected by many things, some of which we are able to control or influence. For example, the positioning of the person we are assessing needs to be considered (will the person be in bed, in a wheelchair, a standing frame or perhaps even a hydrotherapy pool? What is the impact of these different positions and environments?).

3.6 Sensory functioning

Sensory assessments are often contributed to by many members of the team but gathering information from all and considering the impact of this information on a person's ability to be aware of and/or respond to stimuli is crucial. We are looking for both where difficulties and opportunities lie. This is illustrated in Table 3.1.

3.7 Motor

We need to think about how to manage assessment in the context of specific motor difficulties such as hemiplegia, tetraplegia, contractures, spasticity, subluxed shoulder, or heterotopic ossification. We need to consider how physical disabilities are impacting the range of movement, and how the impact of pain and medication on these factors and cognitive impairment may influence it (i.e. dyspraxia). Although this information is likely to have

Table 3.1 What the team looks for when exploring sensory function

Vision	Check functional vision – can the person see and/or make sense of what they see? Check for: • Blindness • Diplopia • Hemianopia • Inattention • Nystagmus • Visuospatial • Use/need glasses • Age-related vision changes
Hearing	What is the evidence that the person is hearing? Check: • Both ears – you may need to present from one side. • Are hearing aids worn and if so are they charged and appropriately adjusted? • Are they experiencing tinnitus? • Is there a need to manage other environmental sound?
Vestibular	Check vestibular function. Does the person feel: • Lightheaded • Dizzy • Off balance Look for clues in e.g. nystagmus Consider a whether a specialist audiovestibular assessment is required
Touch	Is tactile sensation absent, or does the person have poor sensation or altered sensation? Are there body schema changes? Is the person's proprioception intact? Do you need to consider the impact of phantom limb phenomena? Might they be experiencing • Numbness/tingling? • Hypersensitivity? • Pain?
Taste	Can the person taste? Have there been changes in preferences for tastes?[a] Is taste enjoyable and reinforcing?[b] –
Smell	Is the person anosomic? If the person has a tracheostomy is limited air through the nostrils limiting the ability to smell? Have there been changes in preferences for smells?[a]

[a] Just because a person enjoyed a particular taste/smell before their brain injury does not mean that will be the case after their brain injury. Olfaction is commonly impaired in traumatic brain injury, known as anosmia.
[b] Products such as Biozoon may be helpful where this is the case but swallowing is an issue.

been described by the team, we need to consider what we can use or what we should not try as part of a wider assessment of behaviour and cognition. As mentioned before, we need to think in the broadest terms of what might be the reason for a motor response or what might be the reason that we see no response, and we then need to test these hypotheses.

Sometimes patterns of movements can be set up by positional changes, and these patterns might interfere with a functional response and indeed might be misinterpreted and delay or change the nature of a response from those working with the person. For example, a patient who was referred for assistance to manage a challenging behaviour because it was reported that when she was positioned in bed in the evening, she would kick out inadvertently striking staff and would not sleep. In conversation with the physiotherapist, it was discovered that injuries to her back and surgical treatment of these in the original accident alongside a shortening of her abdominal muscles meant that lying flat would be uncomfortable for this patient and that more likely than not an abnormal movement pattern could be triggered. The 'kicking out' stopped completely by slightly raising the back of the bed and so reducing the stretch on this person when lying flat and interrupting the movement pattern. There are also frequent examples of repetitive circling of the arms in patients which interfere with feeding and are sometimes interpreted as the patient pushing the food away when in fact the movement may be more of a righting reflex in a person with vestibular difficulties who is feeling like they are falling. As neuropsychologists, we are taught to consider what a person may be trying to communicate with a behaviour or more broadly what the function of a behaviour might be. As scientist practitioners, we need to consider this as broadly as possible and to test our hypotheses, not necessarily to assume that this has been done when we are sent referrals with information that suggests that a behaviour might have a specific intent.

It may also be the case that careful positioning enables a person to produce a movement that might be functional, but which they are not able to do without such careful positioning. This might be at a very basic level, such as supporting an arm on a wheelchair tray with towels, enabling a patient to use a switch or a call bell. Or it may be more complex, using specialist equipment to enable a functional movement. Of course, a difficulty executing a movement may not be a consequence of sensory or motor impairment but rather a consequence of cognitive impairments in initiation, dyspraxia, perseveration for example. Where dyspraxia is a known difficulty, therapeutic techniques may include hand-over-hand facilitation by the therapist. This enables a person to be supported to initiate getting a movement started, with the argument being that once a motor programme has begun, the movement can be achieved successfully. Similar arguments are employed when a person has difficulty initiating activity. However, using a movement that is supported as a response to an assessment question should alert some concerns. We have seen such methods used by teams who are keen to try to find a way to 'unlock communication' for a person, and it is very seductive to fall into the trap of proving what you hope to see, rather than testing the null hypothesis. For example, a team may believe that a person uses a particular head movement to indicate 'yes', and they may assess this by holding the person's head. However, unless this is properly tested and the team member providing the support to the movement is unable to hear the question asked or see the faces of the patient or the other therapists, a true blind study or method is not valid.

3.8 Communicative

Clearly, consideration of communication and communicative intent is needed in making our assessments. At a basic level, one might start with receptive language or comprehension and the factors that might affect this including attention, sensory changes, and so on. Can the person follow commands? Can they answer questions, regardless of whether their answers are right or wrong? We need to consider their expressive communication, whether they are able to express themselves verbally, whether their expressive language is accurate or understandable, if not verbal do they have another means of expressing a response? Can they use language but not speech and if so, what tools might assist them in doing so? Assumptions are often made that technology can solve communication problems but however good it is, technology cannot be used by all, and eye gaze technology may not be the answer for cognitive, sensory or motor difficulty reasons.

Aphasia is likely to limit a person's ability to understand questions, instructions, or descriptions. Speech and language therapy colleagues may well have conducted a detailed assessment of the nature of aphasic difficulties and have produced guidelines to support communication or be working on a specific rehabilitation programme to address the aphasia. Discussions with these colleagues are of importance.

3.9 Building the assessment

Having considered the available information, one is left with the question of where to start. If you walk onto a ward, into a care home or into someone's own home, what will you do first? The rule of thumb is to consider each naturalistic, normal interaction as an opportunity to observe and assess behaviours. This personalised approach starts from the first interaction. Approaching someone (visual field), waving hello (visual cue), and saying hello (verbal cue) offers the first opportunity to check whether a person can see, track, hear, reciprocate a social response and/or show communicative intent. For example, when we knock on the patient's door, we observe if there is a response, and this affects what we do next. In the absence of any response, we are likely to try walking into the patient's eye line and observing if their eyes look towards us – do they track our movements, do they track past their midline or focus their eyes on an object we present to them? Is there a difference if we show them a mirror and see if they can follow this with their eyes? Do they respond to a sudden loud noise? If the patient initially looks towards the source of the sound when we knock, then we will see how they react to greetings and questions. Can they look at a target object from a choice of two (preferably using their own items as these potentially hold higher meaning for the patient)? If we show them some photographs, can they look at the correct family member when asked to do so? If the photo is presented upside down do they turn it to the correct orientation? If they respond to the initial knock with a verbalisation (e.g. they say 'hello') then can they answer simple questions? This process is less about prescriptive tasks, and more about gathering and using each piece of information you acquire to start formulating and inform each next step in the assessment process.

Obviously, it might not be possible to glean all this information at once, but it does provide information from which one can start to set up and test hypotheses about a person's abilities. We are aiming to create a personalised and systematic assessment that is informed by neuroanatomical, neuro-pathological, neuropsychological, and statistical approaches to structured behavioural-based assessment. We need to create hypotheses that it is possible to test and we need to consider the following:

1 Do not make any assumptions about the most basic underlying senses (such as vision and hearing) or cognitive skills
2 Examine what is known about the mechanism of how the brain was damaged
3 Examine what is known about the neuroanatomical changes
4 Examine what is known about the interventions to the brain in the acute phases
5 Determine the person's medical wellness – people may have infections (chest, UTI), pressure areas and be unwell
6 Examine what medications the person is taking that could impact on arousal and cognition (for example, some epileptic medications dampen down electrical activity in the brain without discriminating between helpful activity and unhelpful epileptiform activity. Some muscle spasticity medications have cognitive slowing effects)
7 Consider what is known about the impact of fatigue and energy management in brain injury in general and how that may be important in the assessment (for example, if the nursing team are getting the person washed, dressed, attaching feed, administering medications, hoisting, transferring the person into the wheelchair for your session, the person may already have experienced sensory overload with the handling and activity and be very fatigued)
8 Consider what is known about the impact of brain injury on speed of information processing and attentional control (if you have to see them in bed, what can you control to reduce demands?)

9   Remember assessment is effortful for the person, prioritise what is important to know
10   Use structured behavioural-based observations. What is known about the person at rest without any interaction, what range of sounds and movements occur spontaneously and naturally? It is critical not to over interpret a movement later, when it is clear that this can happen irrespective of stimulus. Be able to differentiate between reflexive responses and purposeful (and therefore meaningful responses).
11   Examine for patterns of performance consistent with known patterns seen within a clinical population

What we hope is illustrated in this chapter so far, is that (a) structured, replicable, and detailed assessments are still important when there is global and profound brain injury; (b) this is not using standardised tests designed for other clinical populations; (c) that complex neuro-disability challenges clinicians to shift the paradigm of how assessment is approached; (d) the importance of gathering information about all the different domains and using this information when planning and conducting our own assessments. In a rehabilitation centre, one may have information from others in the team but when working with someone who does not have other therapy staff involved, information may be very sparse; and (e) the information gained from assessment is used to create a formulation, and Chapter 7 describes this process in more detail. The next chapters describe considerations in assessment of cognition, mood, and behaviour in more depth.

3.10 Clinical considerations in the design of neurorehabilitation interventions for people with complex neuro-disability

For those with the most severe impairments, such as those in PDOC, an active rehabilitation process is not possible, and the approach taken with such patients is generally referred to as 'disability management' rather than 'neurorehabilitation'. For those who have emerged and people with complex neuro-disability, a programme that deals with both active rehabilitation goals and disability management is needed. This should manage both aspects whilst keeping the programme person-centred requiring high levels of coordination, particularly since there is likely to be a large number of team members involved. Although there is a wide range of evidence-based interventions used with clients in other neurorehabilitation settings, many of these cannot be used with people with complex neuro-disability or require substantive adaptations to the conventional methodology to be successful.

3.11 Ensuring a patient-centred approach

Whilst all clinicians understand that a client-centred approach is best practice in neurorehabilitation, we nevertheless see common mistakes when people work infrequently in complex neuro-disability, or when their previous experience has been with less severely impaired patients. These include:

1 Selecting an intervention that has an evidence base with less severely brain-injured patients, but which is doomed to failure with these patients as their underlying cognitive abilities are too impaired to make use of it
2 Setting goals that do not have sufficient personal meaning for the patient due to the clinician having an overly task or manualised approach to intervention.

These mistakes happen with the best of intentions, often because the clinician is trying to use the wrong tool for the job. The toolbox analogy can be helpful in supervision because it helps supervisees visualise the problem. If the only tool you have in your box is a hammer, then you will keep hammering away when the tool you actually need is a screwdriver or a chisel.

At each step of the way, efforts should be made to personalise the intervention programme so that both person and family can make links between the therapy tasks and how they link to any goals or actions. Materials should be personalised wherever possible. Goals of any intervention should have meaning for a person and should have an eye on the person's previous lifestyle and expected discharge context. It is also worth considering personality factors – some people like to be dependent on others for some things whereas others really do not. For example, some people will really want to master toileting alone and use a lot of energy to do that, whilst others are happy to have assistance for toileting but want to prioritise their energies on mastering feeding themselves. Considerations such as this are likely to affect both the nature of any goals that are set and also thoughts about whether, and if so how, support for adjustment can be offered.

As described in Chapter 2, the legal basis for providing assessment and rehabilitation is consent. When a person is assessed as unable to make that decision (MCA, 2005), a best interests decision-making process for that specific decision is needed. It is common to see comments in rehabilitation notes such as 'Consent for session given'. This can be problematic when working with people with such impaired cognition. For example, a person may nod their head or say 'yes' when asked if they want to go to their therapy session, but this does not necessarily equate to informed consent. For people who are not oriented to place, cannot remember that they have had a brain injury, lack insight into their difficulties and do not fully recollect their previous interactions with the clinician, these responses are best framed as assent to interact with the friendly person, rather than giving informed consent for the specific therapeutic interventions. Similarly, when people decline to give assent, it should not be assumed that this reflects a capacitous decision to refuse treatment. Clinicians should explore reasons for refusals and do their best to ascertain if the person understands the purpose of the session and how participating in it links to their overall goals. Obviously, there will be times when people wish to decline sessions and this could be for a wide range of reasons, for example, they do not feel well on that particular day, or they do not see the session as a priority (which may require a re-think about their goals to make them more personally relevant). However, when people lack the capacity to make informed decisions about their intervention plan, careful thought should then be given to how to maximise the chances of them participating, and this may entail presenting the sessions in a different way. For example, instead of 'Do you want to come to your psychology/physiotherapy session?', saying 'I've come to talk to you about how I can help you with your memory difficulties' or 'I'm here to take you off the ward to do something different in the gym/outside'.

3.12 Thinking ahead

Careful thought should be given as to the focus of rehabilitation at each stage in the person's post-injury life. Within an inpatient setting, conversations about discharge planning need to start right at the beginning of the admission and goals should be tailored around this. For example, if a patient is aiming to return home, then thought must be given not just to activities such as washing, dressing, and mobilising around the home but also to more holistic considerations such as how they anticipate spending their day, what will maximise their quality of life, who else is living in the home, and how will the needs of everyone in the household be met. Invariably significant levels of 24-hour care support will be inevitable on discharge. Of particular importance to consider is any potential deal-breakers to the plan. These will be different for each patient and family but might include practical considerations such as how or even whether they will be able to get in and out of the property, whether they will be able to access all of the rooms or only some of them, what levels of support they will need throughout each 24-hour period, and any duration of time for which they can safely be distantly supervised or even left alone. These deal-breakers are not about the team's views, but about those of the patient where they are able to express any, family members who share the property, and broader views within the family and social network if a best interests decision needs to be made.

Early identification of potential deal-breakers means that these can be a focus of intervention, not just in terms of skill building for the patient but also for discussions around what is essential and desirable for all parties, whether compromises are possible, and what levels of risk they are collectively prepared to accept. Some key principles to remember are (1) no discharge plan is likely to be risk-free, (2) patients have the right to make decisions that other people would consider 'unwise' provided they have the mental capacity to do so and (3) patients' preferences, and the views of their family/friends, must be taken into account in best interests decision-making. These three points mean that if there is a desire to go home (whether it is a capacitous decision or not), then this must be explored by the clinical team rather than overridden by paternalistic concerns. The team must work with the patient and family to help all parties gain a good understanding of what life would look like, what support would be needed, where this support can be sourced from, what the main risks would be, and what risk management strategies can be put in place. Patients and families also need to know who they can contact for help if they encounter problems post-discharge. There needs to be an open-minded approach to the fact that it is highly unlikely that everything will run totally smoothly, and it is reasonable for the patient and family to try out a plan but seek help if they find they are struggling with it in practice.

3.13 Mapping the bigger picture in rehabilitation

Managing the overall plan for rehabilitation and disability management is not best done simply through a list of goals in complex neuro-disability. Coordination of all the different players and their roles requires not just an orchestral conductor (see Chapter 11) but also the same sheet music to ensure that the programme makes music rather than noise. Spidergrams, a type of visual display chart, are a way of achieving this and have been integral in the practice of Dr Connolly, and clinical services she has led since the 1990s. It enables the person where possible, and their family to be able to see the bigger picture, to understand that the neurorehabilitation team is keeping the whole person in mind and for them to be able to link what might be perceived as the minutiae of some of the goals back to the person and their values in life. The starting point in this process is to work out what is important to the person across all aspects of their life, not simply consider functional tasks that the team feels they could work on or would be helpful for the person to work on. From this, it is possible to identify areas that need to be addressed and what needs to happen to address these areas. This is all placed into a spidergram using language ideally that the person chooses and is specific to them rather than discipline-specific. Rehabilitation goals and actions can then be linked back to the overall view. Figure 3.1 provides an example of spidergram for a patient in PDOC with a diagnosis of MCS+. The patient cannot contribute to this, so it was discussed within the team and with the family. This helps all in the team (professionals and naturalistic support networks) to see the aims of the disability management and how these are connected. It can be useful for the family to see that there remains a focus in many areas and gain a sense of how clinicians' time will be targeted.

This spidergram is useful for the team to coordinate the work that they are doing with the patient and channel resources efficiently and consider what will need to be passed on to the next team for the person at discharge.

In contrast, Figure 3.2 displays how a patient recently emerged from a PDOC, who can communicate via an alphabet board set out to the neuro-psychologist their primary values to move from rehabilitation to living in a new home with their young family and to be able to get out of the house and

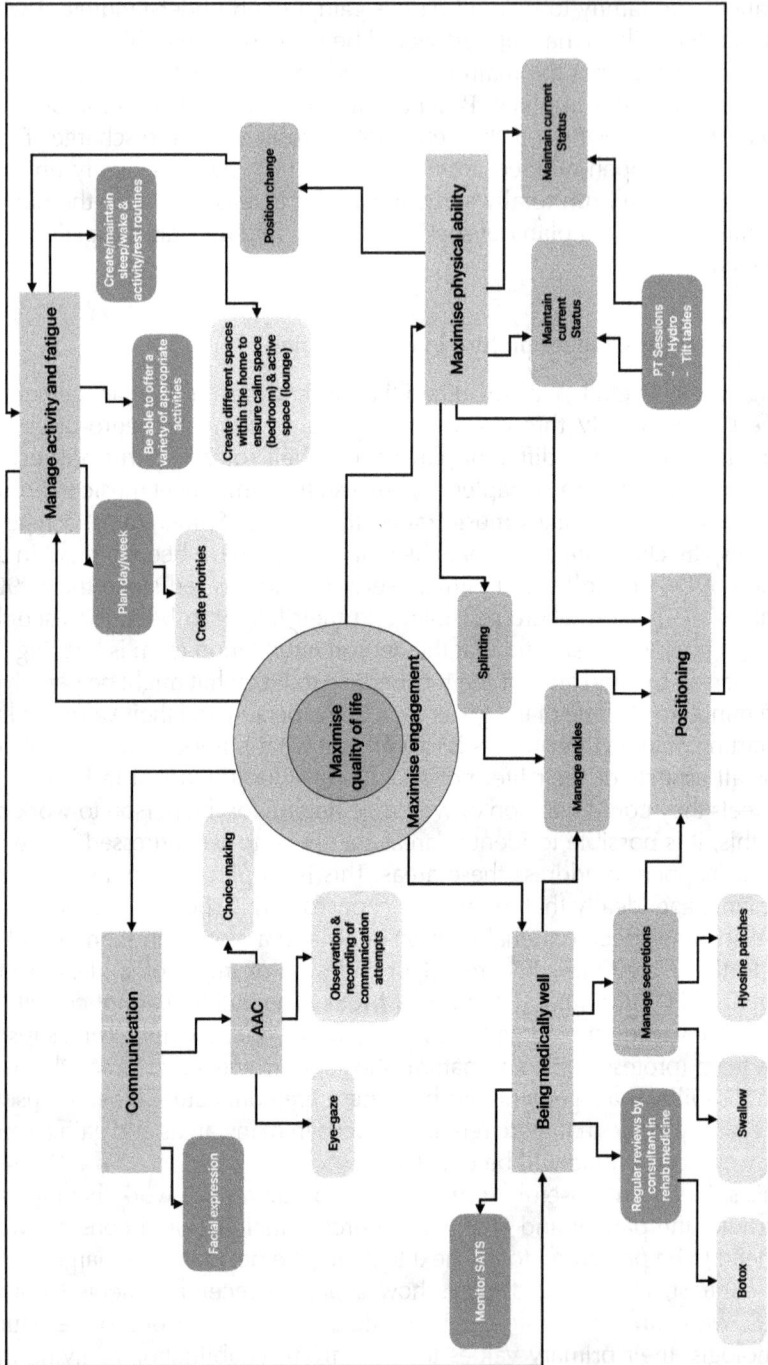

Figure 3.1 Spidergram constructed for a person with a diagnosis of MCS+ by the team and the family.

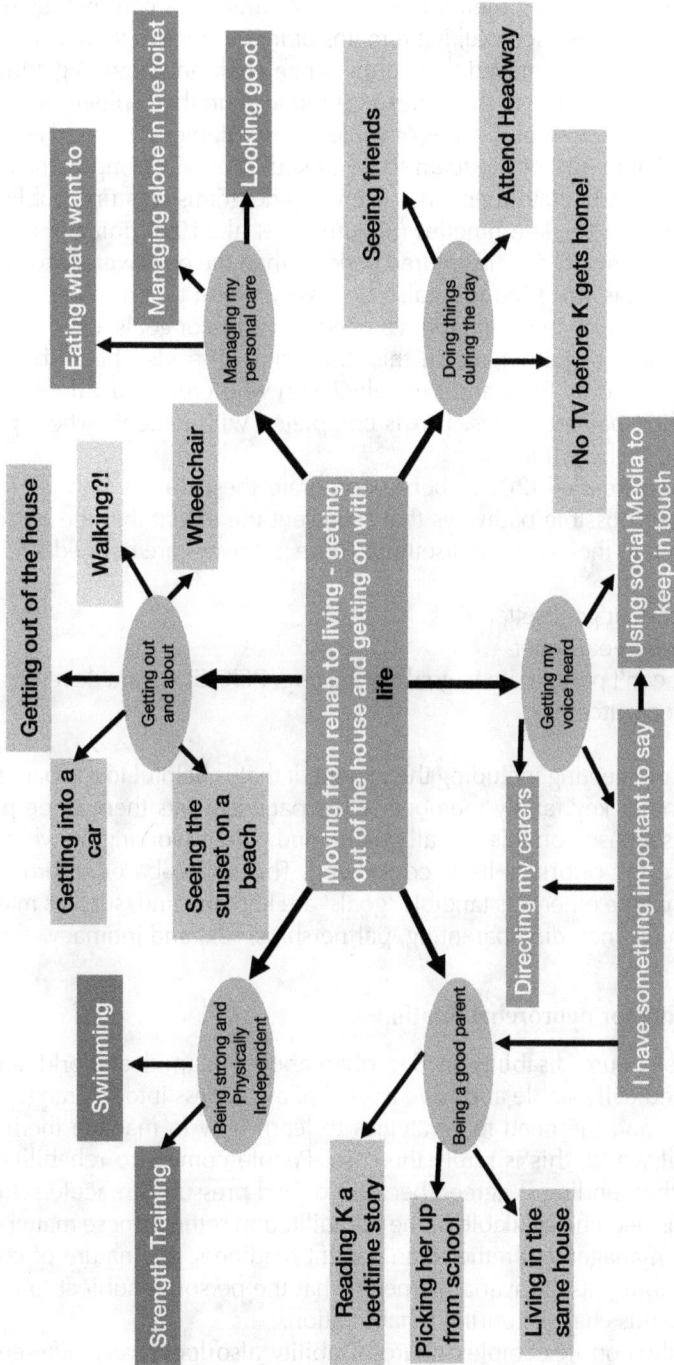

Figure 3.2 Spidergram constructed with a patient using an alphabet board.

get on with life. They still required intensive professional carer supports in the community, but getting their voice heard to direct this care mattered to the person. You can also see walking remains of importance to them even though it is unlikely to be achieved (hence the wheelchair and how to get in a car), but it remains of value to them and so it remains on their spidergram.

The structure from both types of spidergrams enables goals and actions for the immediate work of the team to be linked to areas of important value to those able to articulate them. The use of spidergrams was first published in the literature in the late nineties (Beaumont et al., 1999) initially used with less severely impaired brain-injured patients than the ones we are considering here, but it was since found to also be a very useful tool in complex neuro-disability to inform the team about a person's values or goals, even when they were less able to participate in this discussion. The idea has subsequently been developed by Rose and Rendell (2022) who created a values checklist to help elicit patient values. This is completed with patients where possible and families where it is not.

Rose and Rendell (2022) then incorporate these values into goal setting within three possible pathways that represent the extent that the person can be involved in their own goal setting. These pathways are defined as

- Independent goal setter
- Supported goal setter
- Patient can't participate in goal setting (e.g. PDOC) – team develop a set of expected outcomes

At a team meeting including the patient, if that is helpful to the patient, and possibly other key family members if the patient wants them to be present, goals are set based on this overall picture and who is working on which areas and where the priorities lie is considered. This values-based approach also ensures that the other less tangible 'goals' are kept in mind, such as managing relationships, including parenting, partnerships, sex, and intimacy.

3.14 Timing for neurorehabilitation

In complex neuro-disability, as described above, in an ideal world, a person will be medically stable and have a level of awareness into the range of their difficulties and the need for strategies to learn how to manage them better. In the real world, this is rarely the case. People come into rehabilitation at the time that funding is agreed because of bed pressures in acute settings or when beds become available in the rehabilitation setting. These matters relate to system management rather than patient readiness. The nature of complex neuro-disability itself invariably means that the person is subject to multiple medical status changes during rehabilitation.

Rehabilitation in complex neuro-disability also looks very different from the therapist perspective. In other health settings, a 50-minute session weekly or fortnightly may be anticipated, but working with complex neuro-disability is of course quite different. It is important to be conceptually clear in your thinking about what assessment and what interventions you are planning to do. This helps guide the design of the frequency, duration of sessions, and who else is in the session. For example, if you are working on establishing a base-line across the 24 hour period of distress-related behaviour, you might seek to observe them several times within a day, or if you are attempting to create a matched activity to a person's ability to tolerate it, you may need to check several times a day they are being appropriately set up for this. Flexibility is central to this work, patients are often drowsy or asleep. They may have family or friends who have travelled long distances to be present and all have their own needs for time with you or indeed without you. Another challenge of the inpatient team setting is that you will hear a running commentary on a patient. You will receive more information than you need and filtering what is helpful and ignoring what is not, is a core skill to master.

3.15 Awareness, insight, and anosognosia

Insight and awareness are often used interchangeably and assumed to mean anosognosia, but difficulties with insight and awareness can occur for other reasons than anosognosia. There is often confusion within teams and families about what exactly they are describing and how to tackle this. Anosognosia refers to a person's lack of insight into their disability caused by damage to their brain. People can lack awareness because they lack knowledge, they do not believe what they have been told or how it might affect them, they hold different cultural or spiritual beliefs, or because of a psychological process of denial.

It is not uncommon to see interventions in rehabilitation programmes that purport to teach insight or requests made to neuropsychologists to teach the patient insight so they are better able to engage with or consolidate other aspects of their programme. However, it is no more possible to 'teach insight' than to 'teach memory' to someone. Teaching memory strategies can result in better functional memory (i.e. having a diary really helps, but take it away and my memory has not improved), and teaching strategies to manage anosognosia can help a person to manage this. This is an important consid-eration because it is sometimes suggested that insight should be taught or improved before other aspects of a rehabilitation programme are begun. If a person cannot engage with a planned intervention 'until their insight has improved' then that is not an appropriate intervention.

A preserved sense of self that has not been updated to factor in the brain injury can be significant in considering a person's insight. In such circumstances, members of the team may consider that it is important that the person learns that they can no longer do X, Y, or Z because until they do, they will be stuck. However, failing at something will not necessarily lead to an increase in insight, but is very likely to lead to a reduction in mood. These matters, however frustrating to the person, family, and team, need to be managed sensitively and skilfully to ensure that the psychological well-being of the patient is protected.

3.16 Taking risks

Risk assessments and development of risk reduction strategies are a core skill in clinical practice. One of the challenges of neurorehabilitation is about balancing risk against safety. At an organisational level, there is often a pull towards safety and consequently restriction. By contrast, the rehabilitation team will often want to push to take risks in order that the person can maximise their quality or life, their engagement, and their independence. Positive risk-taking is recognised as important, but it is often harder to do with complex neuro-disability because every choice can be monitored by someone and who is responsible for safety may not be the person themselves. For many people, there is a disconnect between knowing and doing, and in these circumstances being able to test things out in reality can become a useful tool. Risk choices vary by people (for example, some will bungee jump, sky-dive, race cars or scuba dive, and others will not). For example, consider the case where a patient is PEG fed, but nonetheless wants to taste food, regardless of the risk of aspiration, potential pneumonia, and choking, that might come with eating orally. Consideration of the MCA (2005) alongside positive risk-taking needs to be considered. The following questions are helpful:

- Are they trying to do something they see as normal in an attempt to fast track or progress their rehabilitation?
- Does this represent an important personal matter for the patient such as a one-off event like raising a toast to their child at their wedding?
- Does this represent a personal desire for weekly, daily, or every meal?
- Do they really understand the extent of their dysphagia and the foreseeable consequences? If not, is that a consequence of a lack of knowledge or an inability to understand the information or disbelief in the potential seriousness of the foreseeable outcomes?
- Does this represent a psychological adjustment challenge to adapting to disability?

Recent case law supports teams to facilitate these types of positive risk-taking: *'The fact is that all life involves risk... Physical health and safety can sometimes be bought at too high a price in happiness and emotional welfare. The emphasis must be on sensible risk appraisal...to achieve the vital good of the... vulnerable person's happiness. What good is it making someone safer if it merely makes them miserable?'* (Local Authority X v MM & Anor (No 1) (2007)). Being enabled to make what could be seen as unwise choices where a person has the mental capacity to do so is vital in the process of rehabilitation, as it is in life, even though these choices can challenge clinicians and organisations.

References

Beaumont, J. G. (2008). *Introduction to Neuropsychology* (Second Edition), The Guildford Press.

Beaumont, J. G., Connolly, S. A. V., & Rogers, M. J. C. (1999) Inpatient cognitive and behavioural rehabilitation: Assessing the outcomes. *Neuropsychological Rehabilitation, 9* (3-4), 401–411. doi:10.1080/096020199389464

Department of Health. (2005). Mental Capacity Act. London: HMSO.

Rose, A. E. & Rendell, L. (2022) A values-based approach to goal setting in neuro-rehabilitation following severe brain injury: An audit of service development. *The Neuropsychologist, 1*(14), 37–46. doi:10.53841/bpsneur.2022.1.14.37

4 Approaches to cognition in complex neuro-disability

4.1 What is cognition?

This may seem like a somewhat simplistic question for professionals working in neuro-disability, but it is worth considering. The Cambridge dictionary defines cognitive as "relating to or involving the processes of thinking and reasoning". So we do not have a direct measure of cognitive function, but rather we must infer it from behaviour that we can observe (Robbins, 2011). One means to observing behaviour to make inferences about underlying cognitive processing is through standardised cognitive tests. These examine a cognitive construct by systematically providing clear inputs in a prescribed way to elicit behaviour. This means we can make measured comparisons of a person's ability within that cognitive domain, to compare with others of the same age or against the person's own premorbid ability. The data gathered from the administration of cognitive tests can be used in a number of ways, such as to inform rehabilitation programmes, monitor progress (or regress), and inform research. In this instance, we are particularly concerned with rehabilitation.

In designing a cognitive assessment, neuropsychologists will consider different cognitive domains and a general overview of a person's cognitive functioning. This is likely to include memory, working memory, language, visuospatial/perceptual functioning, attention, executive functioning, and speed of information processing. However, cognitive domains are not discreet, standalone entities. They are complex, multi-layered, interactive, and interdependent. Furthermore, there are contextual matters to consider that can influence the measurement of cognition such as the environment, levels of fatigue, pain, vestibular dysfunction, and emotion. Indeed, the culture of the person can impact assessment; for example, if you show an Arabic reader a written chart, they are more likely to spontaneously read it from right to left. Despite this, the assessment of cognitive function is often undertaken using standardised tests where it is assumed that the results can be interpreted as a direct indication of a discrete cognitive function. As Sohlberg et al. (2023) point out, the approach to cognitive rehabilitation is still often based on matching therapy activities to areas of cognitive

DOI: 10.4324/9781032665986-4

impairment identified on standardised tests, even though the focus of the rehabilitation should be on functional outcome and the underlying cognitive function may or may not change. However, even when the focus is on function, rehabilitation benefits from knowledge about the person's cognitive abilities.

4.2 How impaired cognition gets in the way of assessing cognition

Displaying ability through a cognitive test will inevitably require cognitive functions beyond just the domain(s) being tested; for example, information processing speed tests require memory to hold the instructions in mind, visual processing, and motor skills. If there are deficits in those additional cognitive domains, making sense of any assessment is more complex. Consider the impact of deficits such as confabulation, perseveration, utilisation behaviours, impulsivity, lack of initiation, inflexibility, or rigidity on a person's ability to respond to questions or complete tasks. Add into this, the impact of fatigue or mood or anxiety, and the complexity increases. This is true in all assessments that we might undertake, but in complex neuro-disability given the extent of cognitive impairment a person is experiencing, this is accentuated. Indeed, the cognitive impairments in conjunction with motor, sensory, and/or communicative deficits that patients with complex neuro-disability experience may impact the ability of the person to offer any response that might be considered identifiable and reliable.

It is also important to consider the way the assessment is being conducted. If a person is using a communication aid, it is likely to have an additional impact on their working memory. The consequence of this additional effort is likely to impact fatigue levels, both from their neurological injury and the need to communicate using more effortful means. Where a person is unable to initiate communication themselves and depends on another asking them questions, the whole direction of the assessment becomes dependent on the questioner. It is important to not only ensure that there are closed questions that the person being assessed can answer but also checking in that the questions are the right questions and capture the thoughts or opinions of the person.

4.3 To test or not to test: the seduction of numbers

It is important to determine if a cognitive assessment is needed. These are effortful, fatiguing, and for some people, boring. For those who didn't have much formal education or found the experience of being assessed difficult, and for people who are from other cultures, they can feel aversive and emotionally confrontative. When working with patients with complex neuro-disability and neurobehavioural presentations, it can be wise to try out similar formats to testing first, that provoke a sense of finding something hard (perhaps playing Snap or Connect 4), to determine how the person will respond to challenge. If they throw the cards across the room when you get a "Snap" before they do, it may guide you to consider carefully the amount of pressure a person is placed under with a testing format.

People like numbers. Obtaining a score feels factual and objective. But, the number in and of itself is not magic. There are questions that need to be asked about any numbers obtained and neuropsychologists are very familiar with this. Administering and interpreting tests is clearly an important part of our skill set, and our training includes understanding test construction, the psychometric properties of tests (reliability, validity, test–retest issues, practice effects, standardisation etc), test administration and standardised instructions, and test interpretation factors. This is all grounded in a scientific literature and evidence base, with the aim to establish and inform understandings about brain and behaviour relationships. However, it is wrong to think of us only as psychometricians. Neuropsychology is not just scoring tests and looking up which category the number obtained falls in the manual. We are engaged in untangling the interface between cognitive ability, emotional function, social skill, and behaviour. We aim to use the profile we obtain to predict how a person may respond in any given circumstance, and we consider how various rehabilitative techniques could contribute to an improvement in their functional ability or well-being. So, whenever a "number" is obtained, questions should be asked related to the concepts of reliability and validity.

- Do the numbers actually measure what we think they are measuring and do they do this reliably?
- Should the number obtained be considered a discrete number or are we considering it within a range?
- Other than the matter we are specifically trying to measure, what else is contributing to the score obtained?

Cognitive tests are not pure tests of a cognitive domain. They elicit behaviours from which we can infer a person's ability within a certain domain. By way of illustration, consider the concept of temperature. The bigger the number we measure on a standardised thermostat, the warmer we feel. We can also infer what was happening to the temperature by looking at our gas bills over the previous year, and we will most likely see a seasonal rise and fall in these. However, gas bills are not a direct measure of the temperature, and many other things may impact them. What happens if we go on holiday to grab some winter sunshine, or travel for work, or move in with a partner or don't pay the bill and the supply is halted? What happens if we change supplier and get a better deal or if the government alters the energy price cap? Through most of these situations, we will still be able to detect a seasonal pattern in our bills but the relationship with the temperature is not direct but rather inferred and clearly impacted by other matters. This is similar to interpretation in cognitive testing, and it is the job of the neuropsychologist to make sense of this.

Standardised tests are developed on a test population, a group of people who are similar and whose characteristics are described in manuals such as their age, culture, level of education, intellectual ability, normal neurological history, and sensory/communicative skills etc. The tests are designed for participants who match this sample of people so that you can compare the scores you find with the normative data (in other words, comparing apples with apples). However, people with complex neuro-disability have vastly different characteristics and skills to the standardised test population. The nature of the person's complex neuro-disabilities may have led to different neuroanatomy and render them unable to even attempt any traditional standardised tests. In the absence of knowing how best to approach this clinical population, it is not uncommon to see people attempting to use these tests with people with complex neuro-disability, accepting that they are using them in a non-standardised way and struggling to make sense of the results.

It is crucially important that standardised test materials are protected and used appropriately. We are aware of cases where test security has been compromised by well-intentioned clinicians, who have shown and used standardised test materials to help teach/coach a person on the process of testing or used them as ways to work out adaptations. This must be avoided. It is important that any teaching uses different stimulus materials that are ideally meaningful to the person. We also have seen repeated use of tests and continuous assessment (such as using the O-Log for PTA when it is perfectly clear the person is no longer in PTA but has profound anterograde memory impairments) and use of tests designed and normed for other clinical populations being employed (such as the SMART for someone who is not in PDOC but has profound impairments in communication and sensory skills) as that is the only test the practitioner knows for people like that. The infamous case of HM (Scoville & Milner, 1957) shows that it is clear that even for people with no explicit memory, some implicit learning can occur. This means that repetitions of tests even in people who are memory impaired can result in issues in interpretation, and it is important to have a clear understanding of the test–retest reliability issues.

There is a trend towards all sorts of professions, who previously would not have routinely done cognitive testing now administering and interpreting cognitive tests and in particular cognitive screening tests that have been developed for other clinical populations (typically older adults). We see this as problematic because there are frequently problems with the tests selected in terms of reliability, validity, normative data set or an assumption that the numbers produced are a direct measure of a cognitive ability rather than a measure of a behaviour that can infer the cognitive ability, which requires interpretation in the light of other contextual factors. Furthermore, there is often a lack of understanding of what the numbers produced actually mean, particularly when considering if a score obtained is better than chance. For example, scoring less than 10/20 on a dichotomous test is not automatically less than chance. Consider tossing a coin 20 times and counting how many heads and how many tails are obtained, given there is a 50:50 chance of obtaining either heads or tails with a fair coin. At what point would you consider the coin might be weighted? Scoring 10 heads and 10 tails would suggest that which side the coin falls on is determined by chance but might also be considered to be surprisingly neat. Would you consider the coin to be weighted if there were 11 heads and 9 tails or 12 heads and 8 tails? Binomial theorem enables us to calculate the probability of all the possible combinations of heads and tails across 20 tosses of the coin, and any combination between 7/20 and 13/20 inclusive has a probability of occurring by chance at p> 0.05 or 5% and is therefore acceptable as a chance occurrence. Therefore, to score below chance, you actually have to score 6/20 or lower, not less than 10/20. This is something that at some point in their training psychologists have been taught, but other professions have not usually been taught probability and statistics and as a result there can be a lot of misinterpretation.

It is important we consider whether the data collected from a standardised test is telling us about the matter we are testing for, or whether the data is a consequence of other matters. The box highlights some of the errors made in choosing and using cognitive tests.

Common errors in choosing and using cognitive tests

- Assuming any test is better than no test and that if it's possible to administer it, then the data gathered will be helpful.
- Creating a battery of tests based on what a person may be able to engage with rather than a rounded battery, or testing only to focus on the particular area of interest.
- Completing a test in a nonstandardised way but still comparing the score to the norms in the test manual
- Assuming that scores obtained after translating a test into the test taker's language can still be compared to the norms in the test manual and are equivalent to the scores gained by someone whose first language is the same as the test
- Assuming that a person is not assessable because they are unable to engage with any standardised test
- Assuming that floor-level scores on a test indicate that a person is severely impaired in that domain
- Not fully considering the impact of sensory, motor or language impairments
- Not considering or dismissing matters of performance validity
- Drawing extensive conclusions from screening tests – not understanding the limits of what a screening test is designed to do
- Comparing scores obtained by one cohort with norms or cut-offs calculated for another cohort. For example, it is very common to

see tests designed to screen for dementia and developed with older adults, being used with young men with traumatic brain injury because they are simple to administer and score and readily available on the internet. The same cut-off scores are used even though we know that normative scores are different for different age groups in other cognitive tests.

The use and interpretation of psychometric questionnaires also needs careful consideration. Although these questionnaires are standardised, they are measuring self-report (or observer report), which is an opinion and subject to social desirability factors (leading to possible under and over reporting). In complex neuro-disability, if the person has the communication skills to even consider giving these, the scores are very likely to be confounded by the person's severe cognitive impairments (anosognosia, difficulties with abstraction, memory, etc.). Fatigue and concentration span changes mean clinicians may be tempted to administer a part of questionnaire, completing over several meetings with the person. Again this deviates from standardisation and makes interpretation fraught. Moreover, self-report measures are not diagnostic tests and when used with people who have severe cognitive impairments you may not be measuring the construct you set out to.

4.4 Performance validity

Performance validity tests (PVTs) are a core part of neuropsychological assessment in less severe brain injuries. PVTs were developed largely in relation to forensic or personal injury cases but are now considered key in all standardised cognitive assessments. They were initially termed 'effort tests' and described as being passed or failed. Poor performance on such tests implies other data obtained across the assessment may not be reliable and inferences about cognition from this data cannot be considered valid. The premise behind such tests is that they are tests of 'test taking behaviour' rather than tests of cognitive ability. Again, people with complex neuro-disability are not in the normative sample for these tests. Fundamental to the PVT approach is the assumption of cognitive testing in which one is looking for deficits and specifically any deficits that may not reflect underlying impairment. For people with severe cognitive impairment, PVTs *are* impacted by the level of cognitive impairment that they experience, i.e. they fail these tests due to the tests being too difficult for them, not because of reduced effort or deliberate underperformance.

4.5 So what should we do when there is no test?

When there is no standardised test appropriate, we need to go back to first principles. What are we trying to assess and why? Working on the premise that a test is simply a way of eliciting a behaviour from which we can infer cognitive ability, we need to consider the following questions:

- Which cognitive domain(s) are you are seeking information about?
- What are the sensory and/or motor impairments of the person you are assessing?
- How might these impact the person's ability to respond to questions/tasks used as part of the assessment?
- Does the person have any communicative ability?
- Do they have expressive and/or receptive language deficits and if so how might these impact how you plan to assess other cognitive domains?
- Do you and the person you are examining share a common language or do you need to work with the aid of an interpreter?
- If the latter is necessary, can you design the assessment to minimise the additional working memory load and/or attentional impact of using an interpreter?
- Is this the right time to address this issue? Should assessment wait for greater medical stability or changes to medications? Should it wait until the person is able to be seated? Or are they less agitated and more relaxed when optimally positioned in bed?
- What is the best time of day to assess this person?
- How long are they able to engage for before they become too fatigued?
- What is their fatigue profile like – a gradual change or drop off a cliff?
- Where is the best place to assess them?
- Who can assist? – eg. Physio or OT for positioning, SLT for communication etc

Whilst standardised testing may not be appropriate that does not mean that systematic assessment is not. Conceptualising the approach to assessment using the single case experimental design approach guides you to considering hypotheses, methodology for testing these, testing the null hypothesis, and determining valid conclusions. The first stage of designing assessments is to determine the behavioural response you will use to start to make inferences about the underlying cognitive processes. When people have such complex neuro-disability considering this is paramount. Will the person make a motor movement (point or touch or use a switch/button or use eye movements), will they make a verbal response (a sound), will they use words (yes or no; or the names of items)? Will they use low tech options like an alphabet chart or e-trans, or higher technology options like augmentative assistive communication tools? We caution against a commonly defaulted position of using blinking as this occurs naturalistically and can be hard to differentiate or discriminate a purposive response from a spontaneous one. When communicative ability is in doubt, central to the determination of the reliability and consistency of responses is to present the same questions over a series of sessions and at different times of day.

Having determined the ways a person may respond, the next step is to design a test method that uses closed questions and forced choices. Although in other clinical populations the idea is to use open-ended questions and then narrow the focus in line with responses, this is not feasible in complex neuro-disability. When communication is limited, the person can answer closed questions with yes/no or make a choice from two (is it A or B) are needed.

The test method should involve counterbalancing. This means that the correct answer to the same question is sometimes 'yes' or 'A' (5/10 trials) and at other times 'no' or 'B' (5/10 trials). It is important to ensure that there are a sufficient number of trials to determine using binomial statistics whether behavioural responding is above chance or not. The fewer the trials, the greater the score needs to be above chance. It is often erroneously assumed that if someone scores 6/10 correctly on a trial they are doing better than chance (that is they are right more than 50% of the time); however, binomial theorem sets out that above chance responding in so few trials means scores of 8/10 or higher are reflective of results above chance, occurring at p> 0.05 or 5%, and are judged a 'pass' (McMillan, 1997).

Categories of questions should be chosen carefully (e.g. autobiographical versus semantic versus situational) and thought should be given to the complexity of the language used in the questions and any additional cognitive (e.g. working memory) demands of the task (see Pundole & Crawford, 2018). Overall, it is important that erroneous extrapolation is not made from a person's ability to answer here and now, concrete questions to them also therefore being able to correctly answer questions of an abstract nature, and descriptions of 'reliable' yes/no responses should always contain clarifications about the types of questions that the patient has been able to answer.

Murphy (2018) designed the Cognitive Assessment by Visual Election (CAVE) which uses responding by eye gaze (ie left and right, or up and down), with the person looking at the correct item. The CAVE uses binary forced choices (two items at a time). The CAVE stimulus items consist of objects, pictures, words, letters, numbers, or colours. For example, in the 'objects' task, one of the ten trials might consist of the person being shown a pen and a spoon and being asked to look at the pen. Correct responses are counterbalanced such that 5/10 involve looking in one direction and 5/10 looking in the opposite direction. There are enough trials to ensure that it is possible to state whether a person was responding correctly and at above chance level using binomial theorem (10 trials). Binomial statistical interpretation is used to determine the probability of above chance levels of responding, so scores of 8/10 are judged as a 'pass'.

In clinical practice, it is likely that assessments will include both (yes/no and forced-choice responding) methods, in order to evaluate whether the patient's performance is better with one response type than another. Examples are shown in the box of questions in the same domains using both types of methodology in relation to memory, but this paradigm can obviously be used to explore other cognitive domains. It should be noted that in order to have sufficient trials to assess forced-choice responding sufficiently, then the auto-biographical questions will either need to be asked twice (usually with a new distractor item the second time) or double the number of separate questions will be needed relative to the closed questions. This is because it would not be appropriate to ask patients to deliberately look at an incorrect answer. Similarly, for the two types of recognition memory tests to have an equal number of test trials, double the number of targets needs to be presented in the encoding phase of a forced choice paradigm compared with a closed question test. For object recognition, the non-target item (cup in the example below) will be the target item on a different trial.

Domain	Closed questions	Forced choices
Autobiographical	Q1. Is your name Pete? (correct answer: yes) Q2. Is your name Dave? (correct answer: no)	Patient is shown 'Pete' above 'Dave' Q. Look at your name
Object recognition	Patient is shown a ball Q1. Is this a ball? (correct answer: yes) Q2. Is this a cup? (correct answer: no)	Patient is shown a ball above a cup Q. Look at the ball
Recognition memory In the encoding phase, the patient was presented with a set of pictures which included an apple and a book. They were not shown pictures of a clock or a kettle.	Patient is shown the apple Q. Did you see this picture earlier? (correct answer: yes) Patient is shown the clock Q. Did you see this picture earlier? (correct answer: no) Patient is shown the kettle Q. Did you see this picture earlier? (correct answer: no) Patient is shown the book Q. Did you see this picture earlier? (correct answer: yes)	Patient is shown a picture of an apple above a picture of a kettle Q. Look at the one I showed you earlier Patient is shown a picture of a clock above a picture of a book Q. Look at the one I showed you earlier

This approach to assessment requires planning. It also requires a time window, ideally a relatively predictable one, when it would be possible to carry it out. This is not the case with all the people we look to assess. Sometimes we enter an assessment with a plan of what we would like to cover and find that it is not going to be possible because of fatigue or distractibility, or health, or some other reason. At that point, it becomes important to rethink what can be achieved in the time available. There is often a push to stick to protocol and follow the plan as far as possible, but where we have a small or unpredictable window it is far more sensible to consider what is most important. This may involve tackling only one thing, reordering what is planned or possibly even changing tack altogether. We recommend having several ideas prepared. The ability to be flexible and to be creative is extremely important and helpful.

4.6 The new tools of the trade

So how can we work out what is going on when we need to respond to a sudden window of opportunity but do not have or cannot use a planned and prepared strategy of enquiry such as detailed above?

The answer is simply to use what we do have available to create an individualised examination of behavioural based responses. We call this the 'pocket or handbag assessment'. Using scientist–practitioner skills, we can utilise a relatively small number of objects found in a pocket or a handbag, or indeed at a bedside, to explore some basic cognitive skills. Look around, typically you may have a watch, a piece of jewellery, a pen, paper, a cup, a chair, a bed, a clock in the room and personal items such as photographs, mascots, or personal objects that have salience to the patient. Neuropsychologists working with people with complex neuro-disability often have a set of materials that they routinely bring to assessments, and these are useful both in PDOC and beyond it. The box gives examples of the materials we have within out sets.

- Ball
- Mirror
- Cup
- Fork
- A torch
- Large playing cards

- Bell
- Brightly coloured object
- Spoon
- Pen
- Recordings of laughter and crying
- Set of coloured shapes (Weigl shapes)

- Set of large dice

- Thick marker pen & brown cardboard

- Pictures of animals/objects
- Words matching these pictures
- A set of different coloured cards
- A set of different textured materials that are variously soft, crinkly, scratchy etc
- Small bottles containing scents such as albus oil, lavender water, star anise etc

---

These objects enable us to assess at a basic level sensory functioning, visual and auditory tracking, ability to select an answer from forced choice of pictures or words, ability to match pictures to words, to explore different ways a person may attempt communication, whether a person can follow instructions, whether they are able to recognise numbers and to use them, their perceptual and spatial skills, some basic executive skills, attention, memory, and so on. It is always important to wait for responses in people with complex neuro-disability. Their response time can be significantly slower than you may anticipate as a result of slowed information processing and speed at activating a response. Of course, these are not standardised tests but that is not at issue. We know that the person we are assessing is severely impaired, we are not trying to compare how much worse they are than others, we are exploring what they actually can do and any islets of ability that need to be harnessed. This foundation enables the careful design of systematic examination shared above.

Often these windows for assessment occur naturalistically. An example of this was when a patient was noticed on a ward eating chocolate. How this was used to design an in the moment assessment of cognition is shown in the following box.

Input/Trial	Behaviour	Inference
A square of chocolate was broken off and put on the table	Patient immediately picked it up and put it in their mouth and ate it	Visual recognition of food item Motor planning, initiation and movement Positive reward
A square of chocolate was broken off and put on the table and hidden under a paper cup	Patient immediately lifted the cup and threw it on the floor, picked up chocolate, and put it in their mouth and ate it	Object permanence Reward seeking behaviours
A square of chocolate was broken off and put on the table and hidden under a paper cup and another paper cup was placed beside it	Patient immediately lifted the correct cup and threw it on the floor, picked it up, and put it in their mouth and ate it	Discrimination Working memory Reward seeking

Input/Trial	Behaviour	Inference
A square of chocolate was broken off and put on the table and hidden under a paper cup and another paper cup was placed beside it, then the cups were moved around on the table top	Patient immediately lifted the correct cup and threw it on the floor, picked up chocolate and put it in their mouth and ate it	Discrimination Visual tracking Working Memory Reward seeking
A square of chocolate was broken off and put on the table and hidden under a paper cup and another paper cup was placed beside it – But the patient was prevented from touching it and taken on a 20 minute walk around the grounds	On return, the patient immediately went to the table lifted the correct cup and threw it on the floor, picked up the chocolate, put it in their mouth, and ate it	Discrimination Long-term visual memory Reward seeking

This example helps illustrate that everyday items can be used in assessment design and that this can form the basis to generate hypotheses for further systematic assessment.

What we do at the bedside is only one part of the assessment. We also need to consider what has happened since a person came into rehabilitation. Is there any evidence that they have learnt things? This might be in terms of an increase or decrease in agitation associated with a specific task or person attending them, it may be that they take hold of the shower head and direct water during their morning routine, or that they are able to anticipate an action or element of a routine when a previous part of the routine is completed. Perhaps a person has learnt a route from A to B on the unit they are placed on, can find their room, or they recognise a tune or song on the radio that has only come out since they were injured. With a bit of detective work, we are able to start to formulate what skills the person may still have access to and how the team can make best use of that within the rehabilitation programme using techniques such as chaining, errorless learning, implicit learning, repetition, and so on.

4.7 Joint working

Joint working with other clinicians is paramount in assessment, formulation, and intervention with this group of people. Neuropsychologists pop up in the planned sessions of all other clinicians and therapists from time to time, sometimes to work jointly on a goal and sometimes to observe the patient in a particular environment. Direct observation is not a passive activity in this context, but rather one of active data gathering, hypothesis forming and testing and comparison across sessions, therapists, times of day, and so on. Moving in and out of sessions with several other professions enables us also to make comparisons such as whether there may be differences in level or length of engagement dependent on whether a person is in bed, seated in a wheelchair, a standing frame or perhaps in a hydrotherapy pool. The premise is to look for ability wherever it may be found and to consider what that can be used for or how it can be shaped to become something helpful to the person being assessed.

4.8 Pitfalls to avoid and questions to ask yourself

Assessment of severe brain injury has developed to follow a pattern where certain areas are considered to be of importance to assess or where the tools of assessment have depended on everyday objects. We need to consider whether these areas of assessment do hold the same level of importance for this group and also whether some of our 'everyday' tools are no longer everyday. It is worth considering the following:

4.8.1 Orientation

Orientation has long been a focus of assessment with those with brain injury. This is helpful to explore when assessing whether a person is in PTA. It is questionable how useful it is to keep on reassessing. Continuous assessment fails to address the underlying question of: what is this for? how do I anticipate this person will change? what will be the mechanism of change? Instead, it seeks to assess the answer to a different question – has this person spontaneously improved?

Trying to teach someone orientation information when it has been established that they lack it in one area or another is questionable and not something that would be done in other domains, for example, having established someone will not be able to walk again, we do not keep trying to make this happen and testing and checking if they now can. It is noted as an impairment and managed with a wheelchair. Nonetheless, if a patient has emerged from PTA but remains disorientated to time and place and situation, then there may be occasions when it is important to try to teach them where they are (hospital) and why (brain injury), given that these pieces of information will not change until discharge.

However, time-related information such as the day and date will change every day and thus can't be taught using the same methods. Orientation to date/time is arguably far less important than it used to be because people no longer work 9–5 days, Monday–Friday in the same way that they used to in the past. Orientation is of far greater importance to staff than their patients because staff control their timetables whereas a patient's time is organised by others and people tend to come to them. If orientation to time is particularly important to the patient then learning to use a strategy, e.g. reading this information off a smartphone, will be more productive, although in our experience this is very rarely something which holds particular salience for patients. We would strongly advise against using low tech strategies such as teaching a patient to look at a whiteboard or newspaper to access this information since this relies on someone else updating the board, or ensuring that yesterday's newspaper has been disposed of. They frequently have the wrong data on them and are often far more complicated than necessary. In addition to information that changes, we would also advise caution in using strategies which the evidence shows do not generalise across activities.

4.8.2 Will the person understand what you are using as a tool/prompt/discussion point?

There is no point in asking someone to draw a clock and place the hands at a specified time if they do not know how to tell the time on an analogue clock. Something that seemed a universal and forever skill can no longer be assumed to be so. Who needs to read a clockface if your time-keeper is a mobile phone? Is a clock drawing task still current with a teenager or 20 something year old? Similarly, pictures in some confrontation naming tasks are now very 'old-fashioned' and of items that are no longer seen or the commonly used name has changed in response to shifts in culture or society.

4.8.3 Make use of old knowledge when constructing compensatory strategies

Minimising new learning is helpful. Don't be swayed into using 'standard items' where it is possible to use items the person is familiar with or used to using. For example, there might be a view that purchasing a new phone with a certain layout or functions would be helpful but this will require new learning whereas they know how to use the one they have, even if it is now an old model with less functionality. By contrast it is also important to check that a person is able to use strategies or devices that they used before, or that you are teaching them, and not make assumptions that they can.

4.8.4 Using Apps

There are now some great Apps available to use on various devices. However, it is important to consider them carefully before advising a person to use them. Matters to consider relate to the accessibility of the App, the likelihood that it does what it says it does, the impact of using it for a person with limited resources where it is important to consider fatigue levels, prioritisation of available rehabilitation time, focus of rehabilitation and so on. As with other devices it is important to check whether a person is able to use an App and whether it is a valuable exercise to teach them if they do not. Do not assume that any skill learnt on an App will generalise to other aspects of life so it is worth considering very carefully how you think its use will benefit them and then checking that this is actually so. If a person is working with minimal resources, it is important that each demand on those resources has earned its place.

4.8.5 *Recording the patient's day*

There are lots of options for recording what has happened over the course of the day, but one needs to question what the purpose of such recordings might be and whether the person actually wants to keep a diary of some sort. It is often assumed that keeping a diary, capturing film or recording a patient's day is helpful for someone with a memory impairment. However, if this is to be of any assistance to the patient, they need to have an opportunity to look at it again and they need to have a purpose in so doing. For some people this is important, and they gain enjoyment or a sense of grounding from this. For example, a clip of film showing a person at a family gathering can be both reassuring and enjoyable for that person if they cannot remember this. Having a system by which a person can record specific information such as whether they have taken their medication, is helpful if they are consistent and reliable in their recording. For patients who cannot learn to access such resources themselves, they may nevertheless prove a useful resource for families to use with the patient to enrich their interactions with each other.

4.9 Intervention strategies for cognitive difficulties

Having noted the skills someone has, interventions are there to link any islets of functioning found and consider how to use these skills to help make the person's world more predictable, better matched to their abilities and to enhance quality of life. Where possible, traditional aims of rehabilitation may also be relevant. Intervention strategies for cognitive difficulties can be broadly divided into four main categories (a) psychoeducation; (b) compensatory strategies managed by others; (c) compensatory strategies managed by the patient; and (d) interventions to teach new skills.

The first of these, psychoeducation is not always recognised as a neuropsychological intervention (Wong et al., 2024). If we have assessed a patient's cognitive functioning and gained an understanding of their strengths and weaknesses, then it is vital that this information is passed on to the patient where possible, their family and the clinical team. Obviously, for some patients, e.g. those in PDOC, it is not realistic to do this with the patient.

Compensatory strategies which are managed by others are commonly used in complex neuro-disability due to these patients often having limited ability to apply strategies themselves due to the range and extent of cognitive impairments. As a result, these strategies are systemic and with the family and/or team rather than directly with patient.

Compensatory strategies which are managed by the patient themselves includes a range of ways of trying to minimise the impact of impairments on daily life. Helping people learn specific tasks or pieces of information, is repetitive and time-intensive. It is therefore important to think carefully with the patient about what is most important for them. In thinking about how to select an aid and how to support the patient to use it, it is necessary to consider aids that have been used by the patient prior to their brain injury, particularly if their use was habitual. This is because there is no new learning demand. If new aids are needed, then these should be tailored to the patient. The need for teaching them to use the aid is paramount. For patients for whom learning is difficult, thinking carefully about how to do this is vital and will require frequent practice in the learning stage. For example, setting up multiple short teaching trials in a day is far more likely to promote learning than simply giving the aid to the person and expecting them to spontaneously start using it, or doing traditional sessions such as 1 or 2 hours per week. Other techniques such as errorless learning, backward chaining, and spaced retrieval are reviewed in a recent paper of neuropsychological interventions (Wong et al., 2024).

Some memory failures cause particular distress for the person and their family, e.g. retrograde amnesia for events of particular emotional salience such as the death of a family member, a wedding or the birth of a child. It can be very disconcerting and upsetting for patients to be informed that events like this have happened, in situations in which they simply cannot remember them. Analogies such as accidental deletion of the last two years of a phone's photo library can help patients see that the brain injury can't selectively spare memories. Interventions in such cases are likely to make use of photos, videos and other records of events, often with support from family members, to help the patient fill in the gaps, potentially access some memory via cued-recall and recognition, and potentially form new memories based on viewing these materials.

Finally, teaching new skills or how to do a task in a new way, is a core part of traditional rehabilitation. The assessment can provide information about how the person is likely to be optimised to learn these. This should include thought as to concepts like frequency and duration of sessions, the number of repetitions and learning trials that will be needed, how learning will occur perhaps using techniques like chaining (forwards or backwards), setting up cues and antecedent controls to promote success and mastery, vanishing cues, paired associate learning (in this room this task occurs, for example), spaced retrieval, and how achievements will be celebrated to maximise the reinforcements for the resilience, determination, courage, and grit a person has to have to continue in long term neurorehabilitation.

References

McMillan, T. M. (1997). Neuropsychological assessment after extremely severe head injury in a case of life or death. *Brain Injury, 11*(7), 483–490.

Murphy, L. (2018). The Cognitive Assessment by Visual Election (CAVE): A pilot study to develop a cognitive assessment tool for people emerging from disorders of consciousness. *Neuropsychological Rehabilitation, 28*(8), 1275–1284.

Pundole, A., & Crawford, S (2018). The assessment of language and the emergence from disorders of consciousness. *Neuropsychological Rehabilitation, 28* (8), 1285–1294. https://doi.org/10.1080/09602011.2017.1307766

Robbins, T. (2011). Cognition the ultimate brain function. *Neuropsychopharmacology Reviews, 36*, 1–2. https://doi.org/10.1038/npp.2010.171

Scoville, W. B., & Milner, B. (1957) Loss of recent memory after bilateral hippocampal lesions. *Journal of Neurology, Neurosurgery and Psychiatry, 20*(1), 11–21. https://doi.org/10.1136/jnnp.20.1.11

Sohlberg, M.M., Hamilton, J., & Turkstra, L. S. (2023). Transforming Cognitive Rehabilitation: Effective Instructional Methods. Guildford Press.

Wong, D., Pike, K., Stolwyk, R., Allott, K., Ponsford, J., McKay, A., Longley, W., Bosboom, P., Hodge, A., Kinsella, G., & Mowszowski, L. (2024). Delivery of neuropsychological interventions for adult and older adult clinical populations: An Australian Expert Working Group Clinical Guidance Paper. *Neuropsychological Review, 34*(4), 985–1047. https://doi.org/10.1007/s11065-023-09624-0

5 Approaches to behaviours that challenge in complex neuro-disability

5.1 What do we mean by 'challenging behaviour'?

When challenging behaviours occur in an adult after a very severe brain injury, it represents a fundamental change in the person from their preinjury self. Typically, the person is displaying too much behaviour of an unwanted type (such as hitting or shouting) or conversely an absence of desired behaviours (such as participating in personal care). It is always prudent to first ask, *who is this behaviour challenging for*? Answering this question assists with determining the legal basis behind any assessment and intervention, as well as the clinical and ethical basis for input. There are a wide variety of definitions of 'challenging behaviour', and even the term 'challenging behaviour' is somewhat controversial. Perhaps the most used definition is that of Emerson, who described it as

> culturally abnormal behaviour of such an intensity, frequency or duration that the physical safety of the person or others is likely to be placed in serious jeopardy, or behaviour which is likely to seriously limit use of, or result in the person being denied access to, ordinary community facilities.
>
> (Emerson & Bromley, 1995)

This definition has some resonance in challenging neurobehavioural presentations, as the new post-injury behaviours mean that the person is unable to engage in rehabilitation tasks and activities and cannot use typical neurorehabilitation pathways to facilitate gains because their behaviours block these. Instead, they will first require specialist neurobehavioural rehabilitation where the focus is on their behaviour and any other neurorehabilitation that can be delivered alongside this. This can lead to delays in participating in other aspects of more traditional neurorehabilitation for their injury and a failure to make otherwise expected rehabilitation gains.

Whilst changes in behaviour can result from brain injury in general, this chapter is describing the range of neurobehavioural presentations for people with the most devastating outcomes and complex neuro-disability following severe brain injury. These patients have behavioural problems with

DOI: 10.4324/9781032665986-5

a devastating combination of global cognitive, communicative, physical, and sensory impairments too. Although some patients may be ambulant, most will require a locked service and 24 hour care with close 1:1 or 2:1 supervision. Commonly patients arrive at inpatient neurobehavioural rehabilitation services having been nursed on mattresses on the floor, rolling around four bedded bays in the referring service, and the goals of initial inpatient neurobehavioural rehabilitation are focussed on supporting patients to be safe to be nursed in a bed, seated, able to tolerate people in close proximity to deliver their personal care, nutrition, and nursing needs. Many may not have an intact skull and be at risk from both their own and other patient's behaviours. Some will be causing harm to staff, families, and other patients. Often patients will have experienced pharmacological restraints (sedation, anti-psychotic medications etc), physical restraints (mittens, cotsides, tray tables etc), and environmental restraints (reduced access to items, locked wards, and close supervision).

The focus is on person-centred care, maximising both their neurorehabilitation and neurobehavioural rehabilitation as well as trying to promote optimal quality of life. With this in mind, the primary reasons for examining behaviour are to reduce risks of harm to the person and/or others, be able to widen the person's world and minimise restrictions that may reduce the person's quality of life. This can include enabling a person to return back to a standard neurorehabilitation service or achieving their wider neurorehabilitation goals within the neurobehavioural service. Interventions can expand the range of potential discharge locations a person can use and reduce the need for long-term specialist care residential placements.

The interventions that are undertaken to achieve this may be focused on the person themselves, but for this group of patients, they may more commonly be targeted at changing the environment around them or the ways that other people understand and/or manage the behaviour. In all cases, identifying the most appropriate means of intervention depends on a robust assessment to develop a thorough understanding ('formulation') of the behaviour.

Methods of assessment, formulation, and intervention are outlined and discussed later in this chapter, but it is first necessary to consider what types of behaviour are considered 'challenging' and how these relate to the risks described above. In very broad terms (given there is some level of overlap), behaviours can be categorised as those which cause:

1 risk of harm to the person themselves
2 risk of harm to other people
3 risk of harm to property/objects
4 indirect risk to the person, e.g. by restricting their access to social activity/ limiting the range of potential discharge destinations/limiting their expected rehabilitation gains

Common examples of these categories of behaviour are outlined below, although this is not intended to be an exhaustive list.

Examples of behaviours that risk harm to the person themselves:

- Scratching, biting, head banging, cutting, or hitting themselves
- Pulling at/out medical equipment they need (e.g. PEG tubes, catheters, tracheostomy tubes), whether this is deliberate or accidental
- Smearing faeces, whether intentional or accidental
- Self-mobilising when they are unable to do this safely (e.g. climbing out of bed, undoing wheelchair lap belts)
- Leaving their environment if they are unable to do this safely (commonly termed 'exit-seeking' or 'wandering' although these descriptions infer a cognitive intent which may be absent in this group of patients)
- Refusing interventions such as medication or washing/dressing (NB. the extent to which this constitutes a risk of harm to the person will depend on a range of factors – see formulation section below)

Examples of behaviours that risk harm (physical or psychological) to other people:

- Any form of physical aggression, e.g. scratching, biting, kicking, hitting, or grabbing at others
- Spitting
- Verbal aggression, e.g. shouting, swearing, or using disinhibited language or terms that others find offensive (e.g. racist, sexist etc)
- Use of offensive or sexualised gestures towards others

Examples of behaviours which risk harm to property/objects:

- Ripping, tearing, cutting, gouging objects
- Throwing, grabbing at, or overturning objects

Examples of behaviours that result in indirect risks to the person:
It is important to note that all of the examples given above may lead to a knock-on effect of restrictions on the person's movement and/or social opportunities. However, some examples of additional behaviours which cause indirect risk to the person include:

- Withdrawing from attempts to engage them in activities, care, or rehabilitation
- Sexualised behaviours such as masturbating (other than in private spaces such as their own bedroom) and removing clothing
- Failure to participate in neurorehabilitation to make expected gains in function

- Social isolation and reduced access to preferred and potentially pleasurable activities, settings, and people

Behaviour may mean different things when observed in different people or at different times. Thus, behaviours such as faecal smearing, pulling at tubes, or exiting the ward environment may occur intentionally for some patients but unintentionally for others; behaviours such as swearing or using offensive language may be deliberately intended to cause targeted offence in some cases but may reflect disorientation and disinhibition in others. This shows how important it is to have a robust understanding of the patient's cognitive functioning, which underpins the intent or otherwise behind behaviour.

It is also the case that both the risks and perception of harm associated with the same behaviour can vary. For example, the risks associated with physical aggression will vary according to the strength of the patient and whether or not they make contact with another person; behaviours such as swearing and 'rude' gestures may be perceived by some observers as humorous but by others as offensive. In addition, there is potential overlap of the risks caused by such behaviours. Thus, behaviours that risk harm to self or others may lead to reduced access to social environments and activities, as people around them try to reduce the risk of harm occurring. There is also evidence that different clinicians may have varying thresholds when considering if a behaviour is sufficiently challenging for intervention (Alderman, 2017). Thus, gaining a thorough objective understanding of behaviour and its effects is complex and subject to biases.

A potentially less obvious overlap is the psychological distress that observers may experience. For example, patients' families and friends may find it very discomfiting to see behaviours that lead to self-harm, and our observations suggest that some behaviours are particularly distressing, for example, deep probing of craniectomy sites or pressure areas. It is also extremely distressing to families to hear reports of the person they love having harmed staff or used language towards a carer or clinician that they would never have used prior to their brain injury. Overall, there is evidence to suggest that behavioural changes have a particularly significant impact on the families of people with brain injury, contributing to family distress and carer burden (Tam et al., 2015). The psychological impact that staff experience when working with people with challenging behaviour is also recognised and may influence their ability to put recommendations into practice. Thus, gaining a thorough understanding of challenging behaviour and potential effective management strategies is likely to require inclusion of systemic, not just individual factors.

5.2 Psychological models of challenging behaviour

Psychological approaches to managing challenging behaviour are grounded in learning theory principles, which are part of the foundations of psychology.

Operant conditioning principles, which were developed in the early twentieth century by Thorndike, Skinner, and others are of particular relevance. These principles outline how the likelihood of a particular behaviour recurring varies according to whether and how it is reinforced. In simple terms, behaviour which is immediately followed by an outcome that the individual experiences as positive is more likely to recur ('positive reinforcement'), whereas an outcome which the individual experiences as negative renders the behaviour less likely to recur ('punishment', sometimes termed 'positive punishment'). Similarly, if an experience which the individual perceives to be unpleasant ends when the behaviour occurs, then the behaviour is more likely to recur ('negative reinforcement'), whereas if an experience they perceive as pleasant ends immediately following the behaviour, then the behaviour is less likely to recur (also termed 'punishment', or 'negative punishment'). These core principles underpin psychological approaches to managing behaviour.

The two most commonly used psychological approaches are applied behaviour analysis (ABA) and positive behaviour support (PBS). A detailed description of these methods is beyond the scope of this chapter. However, in brief, ABA applies the scientific principles of learning theory to an understanding of an individual's behaviour. The approach involves carrying out a detailed assessment of behaviour in order to understand its function (a method known as 'functional analysis'), which includes understanding the nature of any reinforcers for the behaviour, and the environments/settings in which the behaviour occurs. Learning theory principles are then applied, with the aim of reducing the frequency of undesired behaviours and increasing the frequency of desired behaviours, alongside any appropriate modifications of the environment such that undesired behaviour is less likely to be triggered (see e.g. Alderman, 2024, for a more detailed description).

The PBS approach derives from ABA, and thus the same underlying learning theory principles apply. Both models have a similar rigorous approach to assessing and understanding behaviour and its function. However, the PBS approach emphasises the importance of understanding the individual and involving them collaboratively in construction of their behaviour support plan. The PBS approach also specifically avoids use of punishment and emphasises proactive strategies to managing behaviour, including skill building, in addition to environmental modification strategies, particularly antecedent management, and a focus on reducing any restraints that may be being applied with the individual. There are thus overlaps between the two approaches but with differences in emphasis. PBS has been reported to be the most commonly used model of managing challenging behaviour in people with acquired brain injury (Sloan et al., 2025) but has also been critiqued as more suitable for people with developmental disorders than those with acquired brain injury (Mooney et al., 2024). PBS PLUS (Gould et al., 2021) is designed specifically for people with brain injuries and adds cognitive and communication strategies relevant to people with brain injuries to traditional PBS approaches. The PLUS is an acronym for Person-driven, Learning together, Uniting supports, and Skill building, with the overall aim to help people build a meaningful life and self-regulate their behaviour after ABI. This approach involves explicitly working with the professional and naturalistic support networks around the person (family, carers, therapists, and important others) to ensure that all contribute to the understanding, planning, and implementation of personalised strategies and helps develop shared expertise in both the short and longer term.

For clinicians working with people with severe brain injury, we recommend avoiding a rigid adherence to one model of working in favour of an open-minded approach that acknowledges that all models have strengths and weakness, and the key principle is to apply the most appropriate methods to each person as indicated by their presentation. These approaches centre on changes to behaviour through learning. One of the challenges when working with people with profound and severe brain injury is that the extent of their cognitive impairment potentially means there is no explicit memory for their behaviour and its consequences. This makes learning through a consequence approach far more difficult for them and limits the application of many reinforcers. However, it is important to remember that even in severe brain injury, some implicit learning can occur (that is a learning without awareness). It also makes antecedent-based approaches, such as changing the setting and antecedents to challenging behaviours more likely to be effective.

A further significant challenge we have encountered in practice is that the 'function' of a behaviour is often framed as behaviour always having a communicative purpose, and this in turn can lead to automatic assumptions about intent by staff and families. This challenge around making assumptions about behaviour in this group of patients is discussed in more detail below.

5.3 What assumptions about behaviour can be made with people with complex neuro-disability?

Avoiding making potentially incorrect assumptions (the fundamental attribution error) about behaviour is a feature of any robust approach to the assessment of any behaviour. There are significant risks associated with making incorrect assumptions about patients' behaviour, including developing inappropriate or ineffective management plans, shaping behaviour such that it becomes more rather than less challenging over time, breakdowns in communication between patients, families, and staff teams, and risks of overly restrictive interventions and deprivations of liberty.

The following examples are designed to show how the same behaviour can mean different things to different people and why this impacts upon the most appropriate intervention/management plan.

	Child	Boxer	Patient in PDOC	Patient with ABI and cognitive impairment
Environment and context	School playground during playtime	Boxing match	Inpatient hospital setting. Patient is fully dependent on others for all tasks. Two health care assistants (HCAs) begin personal care	Inpatient hospital setting. Patient is fully dependent on others for all tasks. Two health care assistants (HCAs) begin personal care
Trigger	Another child pulled their hair	The boxer saw a chance to land a punch on their opponent	The HCAs placed hands on the patient and began to turn them in bed	HCAs begin removing clothing and attempting to wash the patient
Behaviour	The person's right arm in a fist shape, made contact with the other person's face			
Formulation – why did it happen	Deliberate intent to hit/hurt the child who had hurt them	Deliberate intent to hit the opponent within the rules of a sporting contest	Spontaneous movement. No deliberate intent to move the arm or make contact with the other person	Cognitive impairment. Patient does not remember they are in hospital, lacks insight into their care needs, and does not recognise the carers. The behaviour is a deliberate intent to make them stop

(Continued)

	Child	Boxer	Patient in PDOC	Patient with ABI and cognitive impairment
Intervention	The child is told that hitting others is wrong and they are made to miss the rest of their playtime	None. The behaviour is appropriate to the context	Guidelines for care staff on how to turn the patient safely and stay out of reach of the active arm	Interventions with the patient: rehabilitation programme to help them (i) regain skills in removing their own clothing and washing their own body and (ii) learn to recognise care staff using photographs. Interventions with the care team: psychoeducation about the patient's cognitive impairments; guidelines on how to help them feel safe during care and promote their ability to do these tasks for themselves
Purpose of intervention	Punishment and education, designed to reduce the likelihood of them hitting out in the future	Positive reinforcement and further coaching to be able to do more head hits in future sporting contest	Reduce the likelihood of staff being harmed in the future	Skill building for the patient and care team; reduce the likelihood of staff being harmed in the future

There are some assumptions that are unique to patients with complex neuro-disability. Clearly when the brain is so catastrophically changed, the way the person will be able to interact with their world will have dramatically changed too. In our clinical experience, the most common pattern of misinterpretations and assumptions in neurobehavioural work is to infer a greater degree of cognitive intent than is evident from the patient's behaviour. This phenomenon can also be seen in other conditions such as learning disability and dementia but there are additional reasons why it might occur when considering someone with severe brain injury. For example, the sudden onset nature of ABI means that observers such as family members are used to the person behaving in particular ways. Thus, when after a brain injury they see the patient perform an action, it is understandable that they might be biased towards assuming that the behaviour means the same thing for the brain-injured person as it would have done before they had their injury. The link between brain injury and behaviour is also arguably less tangible and consequently harder to conceptualise than the links between more visible physical changes (e.g. hemiplegia) and their associated outcomes (e.g. being unable to walk or write). Most families have rarely experienced others with such severe brain injuries in their personal networks, or considered how cognition works, until they have someone they love with altered cognition. This makes it difficult for people to generate hypotheses about what they are seeing and link it to processes that they cannot see and have never really thought about. Further, communication and cognitive impairments often mean the patient does not have the ability to provide meaningful self-report, and therefore, cannot contradict any misunderstandings. For example in people with PDOC, there is commonly an assumption and expectation that the person will have no behaviour. When any behaviours begin to occur, such as laughter, smiling, crying, shouting, and moving (as detailed in Chapter 8) then further assumptions about the meaning of and assumptions around the intent behind these behaviours evolve. Indeed this is also true in people who have emerged from PDOC or have never had disordered consciousness but nevertheless present with severe cognitive and communication impairments as a result of acquired brain injury.

Beyond this, clinical approaches such as PBS can sometimes be applied in an overly simplistic way which feeds into the risk of misinterpretations, particularly if it is assumed that the 'function' of a behaviour must always indicate deliberate communicative intent. The following section discusses why developing an accurate understanding (through assessment and formulation) of behaviour is important.

5.4 The importance of thorough assessment

The aim of assessment is to gain a thorough description and understanding of the behaviour. This includes a definition of the specifics of the challenging behaviour, the frequency and intensity of behaviour, the risks associated with it, the setting/environment(s) in which it is most likely to occur, the triggers for the behaviour, the range of consequences, and any reinforcers that influence how likely or unlikely it is to recur that are occurring naturalistically and directly from the behaviour of others. This assists with the development of a shared language of which target behaviours to focus on and a baseline to measure progress from. The process of carrying out the assessment and using the findings to develop a formulation is often referred to as a 'functional analysis', that is, analysing all of the data about a behaviour in order to determine its function for the person.

There is a wide range of methods of assessment, including both direct and indirect methods. Deriving the optimal assessment tools for a given scenario requires the assessor to have a comprehensive knowledge of different methods and the means available for gathering information. The most important piece of advice we can give any psychologist or other responsible clinician working with patients who have behaviours that challenge is to prioritise direct work with the patient and to hold a healthy level of scepticism until all the data is in. Most often when interviewing others or reading recorded entries describing behaviour, this information is already 'formulated' through the lens that the reporter has used. For example, it is not unusual to hear about challenging behaviours of patients 'masturbating' during showering only to later discover infections, or allergies to the external catheters, or urinary tract infections. It is key that the person's own 'voice' about themselves and their life is captured and held central to assessment, and where a clinical interview is possible with those patients who can provide self-report, it is fundamental. Careful thought needs to be given to when and how to do this (given the risk of exacerbating behaviour), and the extent to which the patient's cognitive profile may compromise the accuracy of their recall; nevertheless, hearing the patient's first-hand account, whether during or after an incident, can add rich information to the data obtained.

Any functional analysis and formulation will only be accurate if the information feeding into it is, and there are myriad reasons why misinterpretations can be made from poor quality data. Many of these have already been outlined earlier in this chapter; however, there are some specific issues relating to assessment which are worth highlighting here.

1 Direct work with the patient:
   Direct observations are usually the most valuable assessment method. It is vital to attempt to carry out your own direct observations, particularly in the setting(s) most likely to elicit the behaviour of interest, which often include those in which hands-on care is needed (e.g. washing, dressing) or potential physical discomfort (e.g. physiotherapy). Seeing the timeline of how an event unfolds, including the responses and any absence of responses from the patient, carers, and others with your own eyes is invaluable, and if there are opportunities to talk through your observations

with the other people who were present then this further enriches the information you have gleaned and provides a chance to challenge any of your own biases in interpretation.

The choice of how to record observations (e.g. tick charts, ABCs, detailed prose descriptions) will vary depending on factors such as the frequency of behaviours, what information is known already, and the preference of the clinician – there is not necessarily a 'right' or 'wrong' answer to this. A detailed description of all of the potential methods available is beyond the scope of this chapter but can be accessed in sources specifically devoted to challenging behaviour (e.g. Alderman & Worthington, 2024). Nevertheless, there are sometimes challenges with obtaining good direct observation data. For example, if the behaviour is low frequency, then it may prove difficult to observe it directly and the issue of using clinician time effectively may prevent repeat attempts. There is also a chance that the patient (and the staff) may behave differently when the psychologist is present in the interaction from how they typically behave, as the presence of a new person changes the environment. In these circumstances, there may nevertheless be opportunities to observe good and less optimal staff working, and potentially to carry out behavioural experiments to test hypotheses. It is useful to ask the staff to rate if it was a typical day or better or worse than usual in their view. If staff report that the patient's behaviour is radically different from usual, then some creative thinking may be needed around how to carry out observations less obtrusively without compromising ethically good practice. Interviewing the patient can also be a useful source of information for those patients who can engage with this.

3 Setting up a trainee or assistant to carry out direct observations:
Setting up a trainee clinical psychologist, assistant psychologist, rehabilitation assistant, or therapy assistant to carry out direct observations can be an economically efficient means of gaining good quality assessment data. However, it is important to ensure that adequate training is provided around what they need to do and potentially around how to protect their own safety when the behaviour carries risk of harm to others. It is also important to set clear expectations and boundaries around their role, both to prevent them from working outside the limits of their knowledge and skills, and to prevent other staff from expecting this – e.g. seeing the assistant as 'the psychologist'. With these cautions in mind, it is nevertheless possible, particularly with psychology staff, to give them training to be able to test hypotheses during the assessment process, to help inform the formulation in parallel.

4 Gleaning information from generic clinical record entries:
Given the challenging behaviour after a severe brain injury is new for the person, a detailed understanding about the nature of the brain injury and any imaging scans (gain neuropathological and neuroanatomical information), the observations that have been made about the expected cognitive

changes that could result from that type of insult (hypothesised neuro-psychological impairments associated and neuroregulatory impairments), the range of medications (and their side effects on cognition), comorbid conditions such as epilepsy, spasticity and the treatments for these that could impact on cognition, premorbid factors, and history that could be important and any information on how these things were managed prior to your assessment (such as 1;1 staffing, restraints – physical and chemical etc) are critical.

Reading and collating information about behaviour from generic clinical record entries can be a valuable source of information, although there are both pros and cons. On the plus side, because there is a requirement for all staff to complete these records, they can provide a good overview of behaviour from across the entire team and help pinpoint times of day or environments not just in which challenging behaviour tends to occur, but also when the patient is most likely to be content or actively engaged in activities. The downsides of this method include it being potentially time-consuming to read and collate material, the likelihood that some staff will have written more than others, and that generic entries may lack detail. There is also the challenge that staff may complete a set of records at the end of a shift rather than writing each one contemporaneously, which risks behaviour being under-reported and/or minimised. Commonly staff will record their interpretation of the behaviour rather than a direct observation (for example, 'John got frustrated and aggressively threw things at staff' as opposed to 'After finishing lunch, John picked up the plate with this right hand and then looked around to his right and threw the plate towards the right where it hit the office window') and it can be difficult to decode what was witnessed and experienced. In addition, when using this method, it is important to verify whether other records exist elsewhere, e.g. paper ABC records, bedside observations or Datix reports, to ensure that this data is not missed.

5 Gleaning information from families:
   Interviewing families can provide useful information on whether behaviours occur in the same way with familiar people as they do with strangers in the person's new life (the staff and other patients and visitors). Whilst many challenging behaviours may be less likely to occur with family, it is important to be open-minded to the possibility that the opposite may be true and to avoid prejudging the formulation. Family reports are particularly helpful in providing context for changes in behaviour before and after injury. Whilst it is to be expected that anyone with severe brain injury is likely to show changes in their behaviour subsequent to their injury, family can neverthe-less give context to whether they are seeing an exaggeration of previously typical behaviour for that person, or whether it is completely different from how they would have behaved previously. This information is helpful both for the formulation and for providing context for how important changing the behaviour is likely to be for both the patient and family.

6 Gleaning information from staff:

Within an inpatient setting, a large number of different staff are likely to work with the patient. Staff are often the people who first encounter the patient's challenging behaviour, and inevitably form their own hypotheses about it, which may differ across the team. In addition to the challenge of staff frequently recording information in language which infers meaning/ intent rather than simply describing the behaviour, other common issues we encounter include the use of euphemisms or vague terms such as 'bad language' or 'inappropriate behaviour'. Training sessions for staff are likely to be essential on an ongoing basis to ensure that everyone understands why specific information is needed and to ensure that everyone is using the same terminology in the same way. For example, we have found that if we ask a staff team to explain what they mean by a commonly used word such as "agitation" then each person gives a different explanation – and the process of demonstrating this enables the team to realise why this is a problem when we're trying to understand the patient's behaviour and monitor any changes over time.

It is important to try to understand what behavioural information is required. ABC charts can often be assumed to be the method of choice for recording information about behaviour. For example, commissioners or continuing healthcare assessors often request ABC charts. Recording accurate and useful information on ABC charts is a skilled task which also requires a high level of proficiency in English. It is unrealistic to expect staff who are frequently under a great deal of time-pressure and who may have had limited schooling, or for whom English is an additional language, to complete detailed and accurate ABC charts. When ABC charts are used, there is some evidence that providing training for nursing staff on how to complete them can be helpful, although even when staff have attended such training, they may report continuing to feel underconfident and unskilled (Winkens et al., 2019). An ABC chart is a useful assessment tool for antecedent and consequence analysis particularly in the early stages of trying to understand a neurobehavioural presentation, but they are not the best way to gather frequency data. We also find that ABC charts are most useful as an aid to formulation and may often not be the best way of collecting ongoing data once the initial formulation is clear. In fact, staff often only record new or out of the ordinary behaviour on an ABC, tolerating a range of challenging behaviours that the person does as 'typical' and not worthy of specific documentation. In these cases, switching to a tick-box system that is bespoke to the patient may be preferable to enable accurate monitoring data to be collected. This can also reduce the impact of another problem we have observed in practice, which is that staff become accustomed to the way the patient behaves and begin to minimise the impact of the behaviour due to shifts in their expectations.

When accurate information from staff is needed, if resources allow, then it can be most helpful to talk to the staff directly. Staff may be more comfortable using exact language in a conversation with an assessor who is clearly wanting to help, than they are when asked to complete a written record (this is often the case when racist or sexualised speech and behaviour is observed). A conversation can also help to reassure them that the purpose of gathering information is to support the patient and not to seek to blame staff, e.g. for not following guidelines correctly. A conversation can also help by providing cues that may help them to remember a greater amount of specific detail, some of which may not come spontaneously to mind, particularly if they typically complete their records at the end of a shift rather than immediately after they have observed the behaviour. In our experience, talking to staff either one-to-one or in groups, frequently reveals that record-keeping about behaviour has been incomplete or patchy, and although this occurs for a wide variety of very understandable reasons (time-pressure, anxiety, adjustment of expectations, forgetfulness), behavioural information is generally under-reported rather than over-reported in inpatient settings.

One further way of gathering information from staff is to ask them to complete standardised scales of behaviour. These can be helpful in some contexts, although they may be of limited value with more severely brain-injured patients. They can be helpful in evaluation and quality improvement for the service as a whole. In addition, care needs to be taken to ensure that appropriate patient-centred goals are set, rather than aiming to reduce scores on a measure, which rarely carries meaning for the patient.

Overall, factors that help promote good recording of behavioural data include:

- Good operational definition of the target behaviours. Provide very clear messaging about what to record, when to record, and how to record it, including clarity about what terminology to use.
- Clarity of purpose – explain why this data is being collected and why its accuracy is so important.
- Ensuring that recording behavioural data is as easy as possible in a practical sense. Methods for this (e.g. personal tablets, computer access, clipboards) will vary according to the service model.
- If possible, collect data during a limited time period. It is much easier to encourage staff to complete good records for a short time rather than on an ongoing basis. If regular monitoring is needed, then the psychologist should explore ways to make this easy and efficient for staff rather than requiring lengthy text descriptions indefinitely. ABCs in a tick-box form can be a useful method for this and carry the extra advantage of acting as memory prompts.
- Opportunities should be created to give staff feedback on how the data were used and why this was valuable for the patient. This helps them to see that behavioural recording is a good investment of their time.

Discussion of some of the challenges with assessing behaviour also serves to demonstrate that multiple sources of information are likely to be needed and that thorough assessment takes time. With this in mind, it is important to ensure that staff teams and families are aware that the issue is being taken seriously and that their collaborative input is invaluable, but also to put initial management strategies in place as early as possible rather than waiting for the full assessment process to be completed. Even though these strategies are likely to need considerable refinement as the formulation becomes clearer, it is important for these 'crisis management' strategies to be in place to protect patient and staff safety and minimise the risk of shaping behaviour in a way that is detrimental to the patient.

5.5 The importance of formulation

Having considered the types of challenging behaviours we might see in this patient group, and the assumptions that may be made about these behaviours, the need for a careful and detailed assessment helps us to develop an accurate understanding or 'formulation'. The formulation pulls together the description of the presenting problem, the reasons why it occurs, the factors that maintain it, and it drives the intervention plan. Within the context of challenging behaviour, the formulation is also described as understanding the 'function' of the behaviour. The principles behind formulation are outlined in depth in Chapter 7 and will not be repeated at length here.

In order to arrive at an accurate formulation and appropriate management plan, we need to have clarity around how to assess and describe behaviour, how to construct a formulation and/or a set of hypotheses to test, how to design an appropriate management plan, and how to monitor and evaluate that plan. Although these processes are described under the four headings of assessment, formulation, intervention, and evaluation/monitoring, it is important to highlight that the process is not usually linear. To give some examples:

- the initial formulation might inform adjustment to ongoing methods of assessment
- monitoring during the intervention phase might contribute new information to the assessment, leading to an amendment to the formulation

These processes are therefore really intertwined rather than necessarily sequential.

In complex neuro-disability, the most important factor is often about being open-minded about the function of behaviour rather than jumping to conclusions. This may involve developing a range of hypotheses and then working out how to test these. Some common interpretations are listed below, alongside alternative hypotheses.

Behaviour	Common interpretation	Alternative hypotheses
Dislodging PEG or trache tube	Deliberate self-harm	Spontaneous movement = completely unintentional Intentional dislodging due to factors such as discomfort, pain, itching, or merely awareness of something feeling odd, combined with a lack of insight into the purpose of the tube
Smearing faeces on the bed covers	Deliberate attention-seeking Deliberate attempt to remove the faeces to reduce social embarrassment at having been incontinent	Spontaneous movement = completely unintentional Intentional wiping of the faeces onto the bed covers due to awareness that something is on their hands. There may or may not have been recognition that the substance is faeces and/or unpleasant
Patient makes groaning noises	Patient must be in pain	Noises are spontaneous, self-soothing and/ or stimulating, and sensory-based

As can be seen from these examples, underpinning the abnormal behaviour are significant changes to the brain's functioning. That is, abnormal brain functioning is leading to changes to and 'abnormal' behaviour. There is often a need to consider coincidental and sensory-based explanations in addition to a range of possible reasons why a behaviour might be deliberate that do not automatically assume the person is intending to cause harm or offence or is being 'naughty'. It is essential to consider the impact of common drivers of neurobehaviour such as anxiety (fight, flight, and freeze) rather than seeing the fight behaviour as a sign of aggression, inferring perseveration rather than obsessions, utilisation behaviour, impulsivity, and dysregulation.

The frequency of such assumptions of formulation in clinical practice merits some consideration as to why this occurs. A likely explanation for this is that they are based on neurotypical social norms because this is the context in which people most commonly encounter these behaviours. These interpretations are therefore built into our semantic knowledge of behaviour and imbued with cultural and spiritual values, which makes them very hard to over-ride. There is also evidence in the social psychology literature of cognitive biases in the ways that people attribute causes to behaviour, particularly the fundamental attribution error, which posits that people over-estimate the influence of personality factors and underestimate the effects of the situation and environment when attributing reasons for a behaviour occurring. It is therefore possible that observers fail to pay sufficient attention to factors such as the loud, busy, confusing ward environment (all of which their own brain is able to ignore), and focus their attention instead on the patient as an individual.

Some of the specific issues that arise when formulating these challenges with this patient group are to ensure that possible medical contributions to behaviour have been explored given the limitations of patient self-report. It is key to consider how best to share the formulation (e.g. with the patient, family, and staff team) and how to formulate the extent of risks and harms for the individual person. Psychological formulations of behavioural challenges can be complex, multi-layered and contain jargon. Whilst this is useful when psychologists are communicating with each other, it is likely to be confusing and unhelpful to present a full formulation to others. There is therefore an important skill involved in working out what is helpful for others and writing/talking about this as succinctly as possible. As with all psychological formulations, allowing opportunities for collaborative formulation is valuable, and patients, families and staff should be encouraged to contribute to it (a shared formulation) and be invited to disagree openly and challenge any aspects they do not agree with. This may lead to joint sessions, further assessment, re-formulation, or to psychoeducation about why their assumptions do not fit with the evidence.

In terms of risks and harms at the beginning of this chapter, it was outlined that risks of harm of refusing interventions such as medication or washing and dressing would be discussed in this section. The context for this is that inpatient settings were traditionally paternalistic with a 'doctor knows best' approach. This history means that there can be scenarios where the patient is expected to comply with everything that clinicians want them to, and this is usually done with the best of intentions, in line with a belief that this is what is best for the patient. However, this ignores patients' right to refuse interventions if they have capacity to do so, even if this is judged by clinicians to be 'unwise', and the fact that carrying out interventions in best interests under the MCA (2005) for patients who lack capacity requires a broader view of best interests and consideration of the least restrictive option. The MCA and best interests are discussed in more detail in Chapter 2 but some of the specific issues relevant to behaviour include:

- The risks of refusing a medication will vary from patient to patient, from medication to medication, and according to the frequency of refusal.

For example, the possible harms associated with refusing anti-seizure medication in someone who has a history of severe seizures are likely to be considerably higher than the same patient occasionally refusing a vitamin supplement. A person-centred approach means that this should be considered for each individual scenario.

- Similarly, the risks of refusing washing and dressing will vary according to factors such as the frequency and extent of refusals and whether the patient has additional risks such as skin breakdown, infections, etc. Thinking about tasks in terms of possible alternative ways to deliver care (e.g. bed-wash versus shower), prioritising key areas of the body, and conceptualising washing as taking place not in one timepoint but across a 24 hour day (underarms only during dressing of top, hands before food, face after food, feet as a pedicure mid-afternoon, bottom during a pad change etc) can assist with the formulation but also direct the intervention strategy.

5.6 Intervention

There is a wide range of intervention strategies. A brief description of commonly used interventions is outlined below, along with some of the challenges with applying these to this patient group. While there are some direct interventions that can be applicable, many of these patients cannot learn to modify their behaviour, meaning that any strategy requiring them to do this isn't suitable, and interventions are more likely to be with the staff team and family.

Firstly, it is important to highlight the setting that the neurobehavioural rehabilitation occurs in, should be a therapeutic milieu (including understood models, supported team working, shared principles around positive risk taking and restrictive practices, shared team and unit culture and quality improvement principles adhered to). The person has required neurobehavioural rehabilitation due to the challenges of their behaviour, but their wider rehabilitation and medical needs must also be met. This can really alter the type of service delivery from traditional neurorehabilitation approaches. For example, it is common in inpatient neurorehabilitation that the patients and therapy staff have tightly packed weekly timetabled sessions. In neurobehavioural rehabilitation, we have often found it more beneficial to have a 'task list' that you can action when windows of therapeutic opportunity present, such as noting a patient has finished breakfast and is sitting calmly, which may mean you can sit with them and discuss outings they would like to do that week in line with their neurobehavioural goals of being in more attentionally challenging environments and managing their responses. Or, you may be on the ward to witness when someone is highly agitated and dysregulated and use that opportunity to practice the downward emotional regulation strategies in action with them whilst also providing an in vivo opportunity to model this to the care staff and provide direct training for them.

Learning theory interventions:

- Promoting positive reinforcement of the behaviours we want to encourage. The challenge is ensuring that the reward is sufficiently rewarding for the patient – as they are now.
- Stopping reinforcement (that has usually been unintentional) of behaviours that we want to reduce or eliminate.
- In line with PBS principles, we don't use punishment strategies – there are ethical concerns, in addition to the likely limited usefulness given that these patients have severe cognitive impairment. Therefore, a 'he's got to learn' mentality is unhelpful – they literally can't learn like that.
- Using "scripts" for the staff to use that facilitate the same prompts or responses enables multiple learning trials and promotes consistency.

Environmental changes:

- Making adjustments to the patient's environment to control the antecedents and reduce the risks of challenging behaviour being triggered.
- Ensuring noise, sensory input, and temperature are controlled in the environment

Direct interventions with patients:

- Behavioural activation – because they are often physically and cognitively limited in terms of initiating activities themselves
- Skill building and teaching replacement skills
- Visual timetables to enhance control and predictability of their world
- Repetitive stereotyped tasks to facilitate implicit learning
- Fatigue management and reducing cognitive overload
- Development of sleep wake cycles and ensuring sufficient outdoor and daytime activity
- Optimise health status to enable maximising naturalistic recovery of brain functioning

Work with the staff team:

- Having a shared service model about neurobehavioural rehabilitation is important. This helps staff to have a shared understanding of legal, clinical, and ethical frameworks behind the work, the neurobehavioural presentations (service intake and discharge criteria) expected, and the range of strategies employed to manage these. It enables the creation of the therapeutic milieu and a focus on quality of life for the person and their family. This also means all staff have the appropriate level of specialism to then build from to create personalised neurobehavioural rehabilitation programmes.

- Guidelines for the team on how to support the patient. These might involve a range of individual intervention strategies packaged into one set of guidelines. When patients can participate, involving the patient as a co-author of their guidelines, or videoing them with their consent can be valuable. We know that just issuing guidance on paper from the psychologist's office isn't effective. Working with the staff, e.g. a named nurse or HCA, to involve them in writing the guidelines collaboratively can help. A tiered approach of reading and discussing them, watching them (a demonstration of the guideline in action in vivo is important for modelling and training), and then being observed delivering them is important.

- We know that consistency is important with any behaviour management plan (Alderman, 2017), but achieving this is very difficult, especially with a large team. Just 'handing over' guidelines does not work – people don't read them, or don't understand them, or think they understand them but make mistakes in implementation. Staff may also believe that it is the psychologist's job to 'fix' the patient, in which case they may see guidelines as a way for the psychologist to be reneging on their responsibility. It is important to note that because behaviour formulations are highly individualised, any guidelines in the intervention plan are also personalised, meaning that behaviour guidelines are likely to be less generic than other guidelines (e.g. PEG-feeding, splinting, moving, and handling) and therefore harder for the staff team to learn and implement. Trying to promote a consistent approach involves the psychologist modelling what to do, not just issuing instructions, and then making staff feel safe to try, giving them feedback and encouragement. This is likely to need repeated training, not just to try to train as many staff as possible, but to refresh memories and explain any misconceptions. The psychologist also needs to be open to feedback and criticism and being able to work with the staff team to revise strategies when needed.

- Creating opportunities for team discussions in handovers or formulation groups is important for maintaining the shared formulation and monitoring whether the intervention is working. This can also create a valuable space for reflection and for staff to share experiences. For example, if a patient reacts differently to some staff than others then, there may be some clear indicators as to why this is, or it may remain unclear given the patient's inability to self-report. The group allows feelings and hypotheses around situations like this to be explored in a supportive setting.

- Reframing the problem. The patient can't learn because of their really severe brain injury. Does the behaviour need to change or is it more about changing the perceptions and expectations of others? A common phrase that helped our teams is 'is this behaviour challenging for us? – then they're in the right place'.

- The nature of iteratively reformulating and learning from clinical incidents is important. We find that supporting the staff to debrief after a critical incident, to think about an incident and reflect on it is essential to better understanding the person and their needs. As the change expected in the person is through the work that the staff are doing, this requires people caring for people, and the emotional toll of the work on staff is paramount to consider.

Working with the family

- The same principles around psychoeducation and making sense of the behaviours, collaborative working, modelling, consistency, and reflection can all be applied to working with families, alongside the importance of respecting their much greater knowledge of the patient and long-term investment in supporting the patient's well-being.
- Family members often get physically close to the patient and spend long periods of time with them and spontaneously will use strategies they think will have reduced unwanted behaviours (like telling them off) and can be unwittingly reinforcers to the behaviour. Therefore, family members themselves may be targets and victims of verbal and physical aggression and unwanted sexualised contact. It is important that they are viewed where appropriate as part of the wider team and collaborate in the assessment, formulation, intervention, and monitoring.
- It is important to remember that services are often only part of the person and their family's life for a brief time, and the family are most likely to have contact over the longer term. Giving families the skills to support the patient (Fisher et al., 2020) and manage their own carer burden, burnout, and well-being is therefore vital.

Pharmacological interventions:

- Although we have written this chapter from our perspective as neuropsychologists, pharmacological agents can be very important in the management of challenging behaviour. This is likely to be particularly true when the person is first admitted, as it is often the first approach in acute rehabilitation settings. When behaviour is very high risk and high frequency, it is usual to see pharmacological approaches to managing neurobehaviour particularly as a 'crisis-management' strategy in the early part of an admission before the assessment and formulation are complete.
- Good team working is necessary to ensure that medication is prescribed either with patient consent, or with a careful consideration of best interests when patients are unable to provide consent. This is particularly vital given doctors often feel under pressure to 'do something', and the nursing team may want a 'quick fix' within an environment in which medical interventions are used for a wide range of other presenting difficulties.

- During the early stages of an admission, there is a need for the nursing, psychology, medical, and psychiatry team members to work closely together in the rationalising of the polypharmacological use, and there is a role of using the neurobehavioural data to facilitate neuropsychological informed prescribing. The need for medication must be evaluated on an ongoing basis, particularly as other strategies are put in place in line with the formulation which may lead to carefully titrating the medication off, whilst monitoring for any increased risk.
- At times a strategic medication trial may occur. It is important to have discussions within the team about how to monitor not just the impact on the behaviour of interest but on other behaviours too. This is important, as reducing the challenging behaviour may come at too high a cost for the patient if there are aversive side-effects and/or negative impact on behaviours that enhance their quality of life.

Considering less restrictive ways to manage behaviours in best interests:

- Staff training is needed in order to understand what counts as restraint, how to monitor and work towards restraint reduction practices and the legal frameworks surrounding this (in the United Kingdom this includes the Mental Health Act, the Mental Capacity Act 2005 and the Deprivation of Liberty Safeguards).
- There is a need to avoid an intervention being put in place without sufficient thought. For example, mittens are often used as a physical restraint strategy when patients show behaviours such as pulling our tubes, rubbing, or scratching their skin. However, mittens are very restrictive, as they almost entirely limit any functional movement of the hands and prevent the person from being able to do other basic things they may need to for comfort or quality of life. They can also be difficult for staff to put on properly and therefore may cause injury or discomfort. Very careful thought therefore needs to be given to any less restrictive alternatives. If it is concluded that this sort of restrictive intervention is genuinely needed, then thinking about how to minimise and monitor their use is vital.
- All staff need to consciously consider and document the legal basis for the admission and consent to assessment and treatment. It is important when people are being treated in their best interests, to consider all the options, challenge decisions to confirm that they are the least restrictive for the person and balanced with positive risk-taking and having sufficient opportunities to experience pleasure.

5.7 Monitoring and evaluating

Threaded throughout this chapter is the importance of monitoring behaviour and the impact of any intervention strategies. One of the main challenges is around how to carry out the process of monitoring and evaluating. On the surface, applying the same methods as used in the assessment process seems most obvious, but time constraints may not allow for this breadth and depth of approach. The skill therefore lies in achieving a pragmatic balance and thinking carefully about what information is needed for what purpose.

The evaluation process ideally incorporates several factors:

a what neurorehabilitation participation and gains the person has been able to make (consider staffing levels, wider neurorehabilitation achievements)
b what neurobehavioural rehabilitation has been achieved (consider whether the behaviour challenges have resolved, reduced or worsened, and whether the general pattern is stable or fluctuating)
c what medication reductions have been achieved
d what skills and quality of life improvements the person has made (such as level of community integration, home visits, social contact, etc)
e what ongoing needs the person still has for both their brain injury neurorehabilitation and their neurobehavioural challenges

If the evaluation shows there is little change or any adverse consequences, then re-assessment and formulation is indicated. It is not unusual that having worked on reducing the frequency of a target behaviour, other behaviours seem to have appeared and become of greater concern to others. Involving the staff in reviewing guidelines and modifications to these is important. For example, seeking their advice on whether they can be made more succinct, or whether there is anything that could usefully be added based on the patient's new presentation, and thinking about how to ensure that any new staff are still trained and invested in the guidelines to guard against behaviour re-escalating.

If the neurobehavioural challenges have resolved, then thought needs to be given to a maintenance plan and considerations as to whether the behaviour now enables the patient to be discharged. Consideration should be given as to whether the changes in behaviour mean that this can be to participate in further neurorehabilitation or for community neurorehabilitation or they are now ready for longer term disability management support in a less restrictive environment such as the family home with a support package, or a care home closer to family. In these circumstances, communication about the behaviour and any risks and guidelines is important and thought should be given to the same principles around modelling and training and how these may be applied to the new care team. Advice should also be given to the patient (if appropriate) and their family about what action to take if the situation deteriorates post-discharge. This is not necessarily to infer that problems are likely, but more about increasing their confidence that they would know what to do in this scenario.

Even if the patient is remaining in an inpatient setting, behaviour change should be a catalyst for exploring ways to facilitate the person's access to the wider world, and thought should be given to how to support them in community settings which are likely to be more unpredictable than the hospital setting. A balance may need to be struck between reducing rather than completely eliminating risks, whilst supporting the person to have the best quality of life that they can achieve.

References

Alderman, N. (2017). Interventions for challenging behaviour. In: T. McMillan & R. L. Wood (Eds.). *Neurobehavioural disability and Social Handicap Following Traumatic Brain Injury (2nd Edition)*. Abingdon: Routledge.

Alderman, N. (2024). The intervention model: Frameworks, principle and practice. In: Alderman, N. and Worthington, A. (Eds.) (2024). *Managing Challenging Behaviour Following Acquired Brain Injury: Assessment, Intervention and Measuring Outcomes*. London: Routledge.

Alderman, N. and Worthington, A. (Eds.) (2024). *Managing Challenging Behaviour Following Acquired Brain Injury: Assessment, Intervention and Measuring Outcomes*. London: Routledge.

Emerson, E. & Bromley, J. (1995). The form and function of challenging behaviours. *Journal of Intellectual Disability Research*, 39, 388–98.

Fisher, A., Bellon, M., Lawn, S. & Lennon, S. (2020). Brain injury, behaviour support, and family involvement: Putting the pieces together and looking forward. *Disability and Rehabilitation*, 42, 1305–1315.

Gould, K. R., Ponsford, J.L., Hicks, A. J., Hopwood, M., Renison, B., & Feeney, T. J. (2021) Positive behaviour support for challenging behaviour after acquired brain injury: An introduction to PBS + PLUS and three case studies, *Neuropsychological Rehabilitation*, 31 (1), 57–91.

Mooney, P., Brooks, J., & Diggin, N. (2024). Behaviour support in the context of neurobehavioural rehabilitation. In: Alderman, N. and Worthington, A. (Eds.) (2024). *Managing Challenging Behaviour Following Acquired Brain Injury: Assessment, Intervention and Measuring Outcomes*. London: Routledge.

Sloan, S., Bould, E., & Calloway, L. (2025). Challenging behaviour, activity, and participation following acquired brain injury: A scoping review of interventions delivered by allied health professionals. *Brain Impairment*, 26, https://doi.org/10.1071/IB24079

Tam, S., McKay, A., Sloan, S., & Ponsford, J. (2015). The experience of challenging behaviours following severe TBI: A family perspective. *Brain Injury*, 29, 813–821.

Winkens, I., van Heugten, C., Pouwels, C., Schrijnemaekers, A-C., Botteram, R., & Ponds, R., (2019). Effects of a behaviour management technique for nursing staff on behavioural problems after acquired brain injury. *Neuropsychological Rehabilitation*, 29 (4), 605–624. https://doi.org/10.1080/09602011.2017.1313166

6 Emotion in complex neuro-disability

It is well documented that mental health challenges occur in the general public and across cultures. There are many types of depression and thus variations in symptom presentations and the cultural idioms of distress that people use (Christopher, 2023). The wider brain injury literature shows detrimental psychological well-being changes and increased risk of suicide are prevalent after brain injury. Research indicates that after a traumatic brain injury, there is an increased risk of depression (Choi et al., 2022), and the most commonly reported amongst anxiety disorders is an increased risk of generalised anxiety (Dehbozorgi et al., 2024). Comorbid rates of depression and anxiety are high after brain injury (Jorge & Arciniegas, 2014). However, low mood, worry, and irritability often present as a broader syndrome of emotional dysregulation and psychological distress (Ownsworth & Gracey, 2017). Therefore, it is unsurprising that UK national clinical guidelines on brain injury recommend screening for mood disorders.

Given this level of psychological challenges in the general population and the wider brain injury population, it makes intuitive sense when people assume that psychological difficulties are probable in the very severely impacted cohort of patients too. Obvious changes resultant from the consequences of the injury mean the person has experienced a significant life change, and for patients residing in hospital and care settings reliant on others, they will lack access to historically preferred activities and people. These are the very things that can support resilience and mood in other populations. Families and staff are often vigilant for perceived changes in mood and concerned about it. This can include families' fears that as a person's awareness of their situation increases that their mood may drop as a result. However, the assessment and management of emotional functioning in the context of profound and severe neuro-disability should pose a number of questions about these underlying assumptions for clinicians.

1 How do (largely Western) models of anxiety, depression, loss, trauma, and adjustment which are based on people with intact cognition and who are neurotypical, apply in severe and complex brain injury?

DOI: 10.4324/9781032665986-6

2 How can someone's subjective and inner world experience be accessed by clinicians when the person's expressive and receptive communication has been damaged?
3 How can someone's subjective and inner world experience be accessed by clinicians when the person's cognition has been damaged?
4 How can behavioural indicators usually associated with understanding mood be relevant in severe and profound neuro-disability?

Whilst historical understandings of depression are linked to demonic possession and evil spirits (Babylonian, Chinese, and Egyptian civilizations), the early Romans and Greeks thought of depression as both biological and psychological (see Salem et al., 2022 for a helpful description of the evolution of the depressive diagnosis). The 21st century has emphasised a number of models that encompass roles of both the biological and the psychological including (a) genetic (b) endocrine (hypothalamic–pituitary–adrenal (HPA) axis and the hypothalamic–pituitary–thyroid (HPT) axis), (c) neurochemical models (involving serotonin, noradrenaline, dopamine, acetylcholine, and gamma aminobutyric acid), (d) neuroimaging accounts, (e) inflammation models, (f) immune system, (g) cytokines (h) environmental models (vulnerability stress and interpersonal), (i) psychological models, and (j) evolutionary theories (see Christopher, 2023 for a helpful and detailed description of these). Families and colleagues often tend to hold some form of mental picture of how they understand mood but may not always be easily able to verbalise it. Invariably it will not encompass the range of models above and exploring how they frame what they observe can be helpful. For example, if an occupational therapist sees tearfulness as frustration, they may stop what they are doing to explore 'what is wrong' and see if there is an underlying problem that the person can explain and label and can be fixed quickly. The music therapist may see the same thing and conclude it stems from the significant life changes for the person and stop to speak about loss and grieving. The physiotherapist may see this as discomfort or pain and want to reposition the person in the wheelchair. The speech and language therapist may see this as sadness, stop and use distraction and orientation to the next activity of the day. The nurse may see this as regulation issues and stop and support the person to do some shared deep breathing. Quickly ideas are created in the team, and getting to a collective understanding is important to guide the responses that are most helpful for that person.

There are a number of consequences created by the brain injury (such as to sleep, energy, appetite, tearfulness, concentration etc) that confound the commonly relied on symptoms to understand emotional functioning. Some pharmacological treatments for other medical conditions such as epilepsy, spasticity, or neuropathic pain may have mood stabilising results (Christopher, 2023) whilst treatments for other medical conditions can cause depressive-like symptoms (for example, beta blockers, CNS medications, corticosteroids, hormone blockers) as well as fatigue and sedation, with some medications ruling out the potential use of antidepressants (Howe-Martin et al., 2022).

Neurological changes are well established in the literature to create a range of phenomena that demonstrate profound changes to a person's emotional expression (such as blank affect, lability, pathological laughter, and pathological crying; pseudobulbar affect) and emotional processing (for example, alexithymia; anosognosia; self-focus and loss of theory of mind and empathy for others) and emotional regulation (like emotional dysregulation; lack of initiation; impulsivity; perseveration). This means that behaviours that are commonly understood as emotionally related may have alternative interpretations. For example, intense crying does not necessarily mean high levels of depression and difficulties with agreeing how hard something could be due to their injury is not necessarily indicative of psychological processes such as denial.

We have observed that there is a tendency in families and staff to be able to note impairments in a range of basic biological functions of a person (such as their swallowing, urination, breathing, movement, communication, etc) and despite this awareness nevertheless make assumptions that the less visible and abstract emotional processes have remained intact. This leads to the idea that when the person is more severely impaired in function, then it follows that this would be more difficult for them to cope with, and therefore it is more likely than not to also have a detrimental impact on their mood. In contrast, a recent consensus of British specialists working with this severe and complex neuro-disability population considered that depression is different after a severe brain injury and approaches to assessing distress, mood changes, and depression require a different approach (Rose et al., 2024).

In people with severe brain insults but who have less profound neuro-disability, historically it had been thought that they would be less likely to suffer from trauma responses, as their memory functioning around a traumatic event was understood to have impeded the consolidation of the event (such as retrograde amnesia, loss of consciousness, post-traumatic amnesia, and anterograde amnesia). Subsequent research indicated that this was not always true. Mechanisms other than explicit memory recall were posited. Van der Kolk (1996) noted that a conditioned fear could be mediated in subcortical structures that are independent of higher cortical processes and thus trauma re-experiencing was possible. Whilst memory impairment was protective against the development of intrusive actual trauma memories, heightened emotional reactivity was common (Bryant et al., 2000). It is now accepted that post-traumatic stress disorder (PTSD) can evolve following brain injury through implicit encoding, conscious encoding of some aspects of the event and reconstruction of the event based on information provided by others about it after the event (Vasterling et al., 2018). In the context of the most severe and complex neuro-disability, post-traumatic stress responses are rare. Whilst families are understandably very fearful of the distress it may cause the person to learn about what happened to them to cause their injury, our experience of exploring this with people is that it does not necessarily distress them or ignite negative reactions. In fact, if someone can tell you about their injury and history, commonly it is done in quite a depersonalised fashion, as they are recounting information learnt after the fact, rather than tapping into an underlying memory or associated emotion about it. People's cognitive and communication impairments mean that they rarely will be able to engage in the reconstruction of the event through others. Any implicit encoding is difficult to assess, as usually the person cannot show or explain this if it is occurring. Instead, the anxiety responses (fight, flight, freeze) are more likely to manifest.

Again, in the assessment and rehabilitation of people with such profound and severe neuro-disability, the evidence base for emotional functioning is limited. Difficulties with being able to consent and the heterogeneity of presentations of people with complex cognitive, communication, physical, sensory, and functional changes mean that they are a clinical population routinely excluded from research in emotional functioning (Rose et al., 2023). The pressure to distinguish between clinically low mood and non-clinical but low mood states is problematic, and it is more useful to consider this as a continuum.

6.1 Assessment

Typically an assessment is prompted by concerns raised about a person's levels of distress or indeed by a person's lack of interaction. It is important to firstly ask why an assessment is necessary at all. At times distress can be seen as an important and normal part of adjustment and coping (an appropriate psychological response to a devastating situation) and only becomes a focus of clinical attention if the distress is deep, persistent, impeding the person's ability to participate in rehabilitation, and they are developing increased levels of risk. This is because the person's response is understood in the context of psychological models. However, in severe and profound brain injury, psychological models may have less prominence. At other times, a lack of facial affect and lack of behaviour may lead to concerns of low mood but in actuality be reflective of neurological issues and not associated with mood at all.

Some staff and families are focussed on the need to keep the person positive and engaged for neurorehabilitation and can be fearful and reluctant (or indeed consider it unethical) when assessment of negative mood states is openly investigated, as it may open a veritable can of worms. We are aware of staff who have reasoned that talking to people and showing them things that could make them tearful, distressed or be potentially aversive should be avoided. Our view, perhaps unsurprisingly, is that it is unethical not to thoroughly assess as then you cannot determine if your hypotheses are correct, you cannot determine if the behaviours you are observing are contingent and linked to the assumed stimuli and you cannot design the appropriate interventions. For example, it was noted that a patient was agitated and distressed whenever a hospital drama show was on television in the ward. The assumption of the family and many staff was that the show created a trigger and tapped into the memories of their injury. Given the person had a severe TBI, a GCS of 3 at the scene, multiple neurosurgeries and profound cognitive and communication impairments, this seemed less likely. By systematic testing of this hypothesis and showing the staff and family that the person became distressed whenever anyone shouts or cries (audio recording) out of context that is not linked to the content of a trauma show, but that they also laugh and smile (to an audio recording of a generic baby laugh), it enabled wider hypotheses to be suggested, such as their responses could reflect a mirroring of the emotion, a basic brain function such as seen in young infants.

Commonly, approaches to understanding the subjective lived experience of a person and their inner world begin with a clinical interview (the gold standard diagnostic structured clinical interview (SCID)) to obtain the person's self-report of this and to seek information about symptom indicators of mood states (cognitive, emotional and behavioural).

Then, attempts to further understand their unique perspective on this may occur with standardised psychometric measures (self-report mood questionnaires to enable comparison of this person with the wider test population or 'normative sample') or with informal rating scales (Likert scales; emoji scales etc). It should be noted that screening tools are largely based on Westernised cultures and the varied presenting symptoms that occur across cultures mean these methods are not always appropriate for all patients, irrespective of the severity of the injury outcome.

In patients with significant cognitive and communication impairments, they are not able to participate in these clinical interviews, self-report standardised, or informal measures. All these approaches are reliant on expressive and receptive communication, recognition of internal emotional states and labelling of these, cognition (insight and self-awareness, abstracting and appraising questions, recalling relevant information, holding options presented in mind to select from and weight with), and being able to have a temporal gradient of time (that is to be able to sequence events across time) to name but a few! This highlights how instrumental cognition is to perceiving and interpreting internal emotional states. In profound neuro-disability, a recent systematic review for people with severe cognitive and communication impairments after brain injury concluded that there are no self-report measures that can be recommended for this clinical population (Rose et al., 2023, 2024)).

These patients are often so memory impaired that they are living in the moment, less able to recall what they did yesterday or even earlier in the day. The clinical diagnostic criteria (of both DSM5TR and ICD11) require the person's (presence or absence of) symptoms to have a level of pervasiveness in their life and not just reflect a current, transient state they are in at the moment of the assessment. It is always interesting when asking someone to grade their mood on a scale at the beginning of a meeting and then again at the end of a meeting (such as 'how are you feeling now compared to the beginning of our session? The same, better or worse'), how rarely they can recall their first answer, which makes using their self-report in judgements about mood states challenging. It also highlights that your approach to assessment will require seeing the person in vivo multiple times in multiple contexts to help develop useful assessment baseline information.

Further methods in trying to establish someone's internal mood state are typically made observationally with direct (observations made by you) and indirect (observations made by others and reported to you) approaches. In other clinical populations such as children, older adults, learning disabilities (and indeed with animals), reliance on another's internal experience is based on the views of an observer which may be a person from the patient's nat- uralistic support networks or a clinician. Some of these rely on standardised psychometric scales and at other times may rely on clinical interviews to understand symptoms from the people who are with the patient regularly. Rose et al. (2023) tentatively recommended that two observer-rated mood scales (The Stroke Aphasic Depression Questionnaire and the Aphasia Depression Rating Scale) had the strongest internal consistency and construct validity for people with complex neuro-disability.

Observers of course infer emotion from what people do. In severe and profound neuro-disability, many of the observational indicators that would be traditionally relied upon (such as going off one's food, changes to sleep, appearing tearful, appearing withdrawn, not doing activities they typically enjoy, limited eye contact etc) are of course confounded by the symptoms of the brain injury itself and/or the treatment of it (such as PEG feed, medi- cation side effects etc). Facial expressions that may normally be relied on for inferences of emotional state may be altered (such as by high or low facial tone, clinical botulinum toxin, medication effects, a blank affect, etc) and make this challenging to read.

Observers also infer emotional states from what people may say, which with this clinical population is hampered by their communication impairments, and there may be very little communication that can be relied upon. This means that observers will be making judgements about the mood in the absence of such information and be subject to the biases of the observer (such as 'I'd be depressed if this had happened to me too and I was in here'). In the context of so much impairment (cognitive, physical, sensory, communicative, functional), there are erroneous assumptions held that emotional functioning remains intact and neurotypical, the assessor must be alert to these potential projections of others and their own biases (Rose et al., 2024).

Given the prevalence of mental health challenges in the general popula- tion, some patients will have had longstanding extremely severe premorbid mental health conditions. Pre-injury experiences (such as a history of depres- sion or psychosis or adverse childhood events) and recall of the injury experi- ence (such as a traumatic response) are assumed to have significance in the post-injury presentation by families and staff. In principle, it is always good practice to have a strong understanding of the whole of the person you are working with, and this includes a detailed understanding of their pre-injury life. It can be helpful to question how much the person's pre-injury conditions have relevance now (how much weight do you attribute to this in your formulation? And, who does it matter most for?). What is often missing in understanding the weighting of preinjury experiences in the formulation of psychological distress is how severe the neurological injury is. In many ways, the injury creates a 'new person' and there is little left of the old self. Severe injuries of course also impact on memory. Some people have such retrograde amnesia or impairments of memory that they cannot recall ever having been married, or having children and yet fears about their ability to recall times of great distress from their past persist. Interestingly, we have had experiences that after severe and profound brain injury some pre-injury conditions do not appear to have been problematic for the person, including those whose brain injuries occurred during psychosis, acts of deliberate self-harm, and suicide. It is difficult to understand why this occurred, but hypotheses about the damage to cognition and memory systems seem feasible. In one instance, the person had many, many scars from deliberate self-harm on their arms, and when asked about them had no idea how they had acquired them and were untroubled by them. Their thoughts and urges for deliberate self-harm (perhaps as a result of loss of attention for the ruminative thinking, the planning, and executive functioning system damage) and issues with obsessive compulsive disorder (perhaps as a result of damage to the attentional and executive functioning systems) and low mood were carefully assessed, but were no longer present.

Given these challenges, you may well wonder what you can do. Clinical neuropsychology seeks to establish and explain the brain–behaviour relationships and having high levels of expertise in general mental health, ABI-specific mental health as well as the neuropsychological impact of severe and profound brain injury is important. When questions about a person's mood are asked, the first stage is to consider why they are being asked and why they are being asked at this time. Questions one might ask include whether there has been a recent change in the person's behaviour, such as a reduction in engagement or an increase in tears, or whether the questions are assumption-based. Families are devastated by what has happened to their loved one and cannot imagine they would not be depressed; staff looking for the 'key' to unlock engagement in rehabilitation might assume low mood needs addressing or observed behaviours may be assumed to demonstrate emotion when in fact they cannot be assumed to do so. Consideration of this framework will help to guide the approach to an assessment.

It is important to firstly think more broadly about what you are assessing, the role of the neurological damage, and how to best approach the assessment. The goal is to make a systematic analysis by gathering and accumulating evidence from observers and any information from the person, alongside your own clinical observations. It may mean that you develop bespoke and personalised measures for the person drawing off your knowledge about the person and measurement (Did they use emojis in communication preinjury? What is the best way to present a scale? Do they have a hemianopia? How many items can they hold in working memory? Should you use base emotions like happy and sad, not nuanced emotions like hopeless?) and your knowledge of the symptoms/behaviours they can show (for example, you may not want to track interest in food and appetite if they are PEG fed, or you may need to if they are PEG fed and trying to grab food off people's plates in a cafe). It will be important to track the person across several different settings and different times of the day (Is there any diurnal variation? Are they better/ worse with certain people? Do they show more agitation in physiotherapy?). With other members of the team, clinical neuropsychologists will have a role in developing an understanding of the person's baseline presentation and formulating a range of hypotheses that can then be designed to test. Recent consensus amongst clinicians' expert in complex neuro-disability highlighted the challenges of developing a formulation regarding emotional functioning (Rose et al., 2024). The formulation will inform how treatment choices and intervention changes are impacting the person. Sharing the formulation with the team is vital as part of the preparation for intervention, as failure to do this can undermine treatment. For example, when a person struggled to be away from the familiarity of the ward area, a graded exposure hierarchy was proposed only to discover that other team members were taking the person out and returning them at high speed whenever they expressed heightened anxiety. Rather than helping the person, this response from team members inadvertently negatively reinforced the person's anxiety and reinforced their safety behaviours.

6.2 Intervention

Having determined in the assessment if there is any distress and how it presents across time, the intervention seeks to answer if this distress can be changed. The first goal of an intervention is always to reduce distress. It is unlikely that psychological therapies (talking therapy such as CBT or ACT) will be feasible, as the person's impairments in cognition and communication invariably will make even a modified approach pointless.

In the absence of traditional models of psychological therapy, gaining control over the things you can is an important first step. Taking control of the level of the sensory stimulation (over or under stimulation) and the environment to make the person's world fit best with their skill level and be more predictable and understandable can be helpful. This may include thinking about trying to match the environment to a person's cognitive skills such as providing visual timetables to set out a sense of the day and to develop set routines to tap into implicit learning and help make tasks the person is assessed to find more challenging such as showering follow a familiar pattern (errorless learning approaches). Making a sterile hospital bed space more personal may include printing photos of familiar places (the house or a special holiday destination), people (children, family, friends, and pets) or cherished items (such as cars, motorbikes, special paintings). If the person has retained autobiographical memory to any extent, this could help to ground the sense of the familiar and facilitate making the environment emotionally salient for the person. It also has a secondary benefit of helping staff to see the person's rich and full life, rather than as an injured person with lots of needs. In focus groups with staff, they commonly report that this can be very confrontative for them (Soeterik, 2017).

It is important to consider how to maximise positive behaviours and min-imise distress behaviours. Using principles from positive psychology, such as creating a log of achievements the person is making in the face of the many, many things they can't do can be useful. Connecting people with valued and important family, friends and pets in their networks can be helpful such as supporting and facilitating video calls with the family before children go to bed etc. For people who are able to give some information to you, they may be able to participate in the development of guidelines for staff about how they optimally would like to be supported, do they want the team to distract them when tearful or ignore it or ask questions about it or remind them of their positive achievement log etc.

Very often there are minimal opportunities for participating in things that are centred on well-being as the primary goal. In complex neuro-disability, this is not something that the patient will be able to initiate themselves, do independently, or make requests for assistance with. Fundamental psycho-logical well-being techniques seem to be sensible, such as personalised and meaningful behavioural activation, and pleasant event scheduling. Thought must be given to designing on-the-ward activities and in the public/shared spaces and grounds that a person can be supported to do. Supporting the widening of a person's world again and exploring further afield from the hos-pital/care setting will be likely to need a wider team response (such as seating, skin integrity, mobility, transport, toileting, medication administration times, eating/drinking, and communication). These events enable opportunities for potential pleasure. Supporting emotional functioning is a task and role for the whole of the team. It is a core part of the rehabilitative efforts and should not be seen as a nice to have or bolt on to the real work. Capturing this, perhaps using a smartphone or tablet, so that the images of the events can be printed and looked at again with the person and also used by family to discuss with them can be helpful. This creates multiple opportunities for repetition and rehearsal, with increased cues to memory retrieval.

General well-being approaches such as access to green spaces, nature, and natural light, particularly for people who spend long periods of time indoors and have prolonged admissions are intuitively possibly helpful. Working with the team to facilitate the person to redevelop circadian rhythms and a sleep/ wake cycle is key. We regularly need to question why medications are given at 10 pm when the person has already fallen asleep or why they are fed during the night or if all the turning and incontinence pad changing is required and if the relatively high lighting levels in the ward are needed. It is also key to account for neurocognitive fatigue resultant from brain injury and ensure the person is provided with opportunities for siesta/rests in the day.

Given people with complex neuro-disability have so much handling in relation to care tasks and physical management, which could often be perceived as aversive (such as suctioning, moving and handling, splinting) it is important that the person also has non-contingent social contact (that is time with staff who are the creators of potential aversive interactions for no/low demand contacts). We encourage staff to hold a person's hand and require nothing more from them. This helps the person get used to people in their personal space without it being aversive. It helps remind staff that the 'person' is inside the body that they interact with. This taps into psychological models of mood that emphasise the role of cognition and learning in the development and maintenance of distress, such as learned helplessness.

At times, concerns that the person could be at risk of experiencing low mood will result in some form of hypothesis testing with a pharmacological trial (an anti-depressant, a mood stabiliser, an atypical anti-psychotic such as Risperidone, Olanzapine and Quetiapine). There are questions about the efficacy of atypical antipsychotic medications for people with brain injuries (McKay et al., 2021) and the potential for negative effects on cognitive recovery (Race et al., 2023). Neuropsychiatrists we work with describe 'neuropsychologically informed prescribing' to help establish the baseline and monitor any response to treatment. If there is no change or deterioration, then medications should be titrated back down. This means neuropsychologists have a role in gathering and interpreting the data to assess the effectiveness of pharmacological interventions drawing from single-case experimental design and ABA designs. It is of critical importance in pharmacological trials that there is rigour with a clear baseline established, clear variables to be measured (dependent variable) and the process by which this will be done before a trial is started.

Sharing the formulation with the naturalistic and professional networks around the person can reduce fears of what any observed behaviours may mean. In severe and profound brain injury, it is unlikely that the person themselves will be able to explain for themselves, and it is key that all the relevant necessary tests are done to systematically provide information. We have worked with people in PDOC where full X-rays and MRI of the body have been done alongside extensive trials of titrating pain medication up and then down again, to confirm if the distress observed was potentially linked to any pain. Then, trials of anti-depressants were used to determine if the person's behaviour changed. It did not appear to. Then trials of environmental changes were made to determine their value on the person's presentation. It did not appear to help. The hypothesis was therefore reached that the behaviour interpreted by all as distress was more likely a heightened level of base agitation characterised by loud vocalisation and movements. A further trial of mood stabilising medication was trialled and showed no impact. This systematic process informed a best interest meeting to determine the person's quality of life and if continuation of treatment (CANH) was still in their best interests.

Whilst rigour is needed for trials for medication effectiveness, the principles of supporting emotional well-being throughout each day are fundamental to good clinical practice and should be applied universally for people with complex neuro-disability. It is of paramount importance that all staff consider the brain-injured person as someone who requires a rich, varied, and positive environment and recognises their responsibility in helping to create and maintain this. In circumstances where the person is unable to direct any of this themselves, this becomes even more true.

References

Bryant, R. A., Marosszeky, J. E., Crooks, J., & Gurka, J. A. (2000). Posttraumatic stress disorder after severe traumatic brain injury. *The American Journal of Psychiatry*, *157*(4), 629–631.

Choi, Y., Kim, E. Y., Sun, J., Kim, H. K., Lee, Y. S., Oh, B. M., Park, H. Y., & Leigh, J. H. (2022). Incidence of depression after traumatic brain injury: A Nationwide Longitudinal Study of 2.2 Million Adults. *Journal of Neurotrauma*, *39*(5-6), 390–397.

Christopher, G. (2023). Depression: Current Perspectives in Research and Treatment. Routledge. New York.

Dehbozorgi, M., Maghsoudi, M. R., Mohammadi, I., Firouzabadi, S. R., Mohammaditabar, M., Oraee, S., Aarabi, A., Goodarzi, M., Shafiee, A., & Bakhtiyari, M. (2024). Incidence of anxiety after traumatic brain injury: A systematic review and meta-analysis. *BMC Neurology*, *24*(1), 293.

Howe-Martin, L., Knox-Rice, T., Denman, D., & Sherwood Brown, E. (2022). Depression and comorbid medical illness. In S.M. McClintock & J. Choi (Eds). Neuropsychology of Depression. Guildford Press. New York.

Jorge, R. E., & Arciniegas, D. B. (2014). Mood disorders after TBI. *The Psychiatric clinics of North America*, *37*(1), 13–29. https://doi.org/10.1016/j.psc.2013.11.005

McKay, A., Trevena-Peters, J., & Ponsford, J. (2021). The use of atypical antipsychotics for managing agitation after traumatic brain injury. *The Journal of Head Trauma Rehabilitation*, *36*(3), 149–155.

Ownsworth, T., & Gracey, F (2017). *Cognitive Behavioural Therapy for People with Brain Injury*. In B, Wilson., J, Winegardner., C, van Heugten., & T, Ownsworth (Eds.). Neuropsychological Rehabilitation: The International Handbook (1st ed.). Routledge.

Race, N. S., Moschonas, E. H., Cheng, J. P., Bondi, C. O., & Kline, A. E. (2023). Antipsychotic drugs: The antithesis to neurorehabilitation in models of pre-clinical traumatic brain injury. *Neurotrauma Reports*, *4*(1), 724–735.

Rose, A. E., Cullen, B., Crawford, S., & Evans, J. J. (2023). A systematic review of mood and depression measures in people with severe cognitive and communication impairments following acquired brain injury. *Clinical Rehabilitation*, *37*(5), 679–700.

Rose, A. E., Cullen, B., Crawford, S., & Evans, J. J. (2024). Working towards consensus on the assessment of mood after severe acquired brain injury: Focus groups with UK-based professionals. *Clinical Rehabilitation*, *38*(12), 1703–1710.

Salem, H., Soares, J. C., & Selvaraj, S. (2022). Depression and major depressive disorder: Evolution of diagnosis and symptomatology. In S. M. McClintock & J. Choi (Eds). Neuropsychology of Depression. Guildford Press. New York.

Soeterik, S. M. (2017). The experience of families and health care professionals supporting people with prolonged disorders of consciousness. [Doctoral Thesis, Royal Holloway, University of London].

van der Kolk, B. A. (1996). The psychobiology of PTSD, in Traumatic Stress: The Effects of Overwhelming Experience on Mind, Body, and Society. Edited by van der Kolk BA, McFarlane AC, Weisaeth L. New York, Guilford Press, pp 214–241.

Vasterling, J. J., Jacob, S. N., & Rasmusson, A. (2018). Traumatic brain injury and posttraumatic stress disorder: Conceptual, diagnostic, and therapeutic considerations in the context of co-occurrence. *The Journal of Neuropsychiatry and Clinical Neurosciences, 30(2)*, 91–100.

7 How do we make sense of the presentation?

Complex case formulation

There is clearly an understanding within the field of neurorehabilitation that a return to life just as it was prior to the brain insult is not likely to be fully achieved. Indeed Wilson (2017) specifies 'rehabilitation' is not equivalent to 'recovery'. The aims of rehabilitation for those with complex neuro-disability are likely to be very different, as is discussed in Chapter 3. However, families are usually still looking for teams to provide an intervention that focuses on identifying and mending a problem for their loved one. Bringing a team to a shared formulation of what they are seeing in a person's behaviour after severe and profound brain injury, what they might hope to achieve through rehabilitation and supporting the family to understand this, requires different skills, and an ability to hold distress and sit with so much uncertainty. The nature of these different skills is explored in this chapter.

Rehabilitation comes with a sense of time pressure. This is exacerbated with this group of patients because the changes and progress they make are usually very slow and because they are often not able to tell you about their goals, their priorities, when change is made, and so on. NHS rehabilitation is time-limited in the UK, and the way funding is organised, both in terms of when funding is available versus when a person is 'ready' for rehabilitation (both medically and psychologically) and also how long someone might require funding for, adds pressure which pushes the team to 'do' as soon as possible and this in turn can result in a less coordinated team approach. Best practice indicates the need for an integrated plan for rehabilitation where progress can be measured, and adaptations to the plan can be made in a coordinated manner. Doing this demands a proper formulation encompassing the patient's presentation and how change can be tracked. Whilst evidence-based practice is at the heart of rehabilitation, as discussed there can often be a dearth of evidence for this population and so decisions are made based on the best available evidence. This can require negotiation in the team and with the family.

The process of developing a neurorehabilitation programme for a person with complex neuro-disability follows the general rule of gathering information through a process of different assessment methods and then integrating

DOI: 10.4324/9781032665986-7

that information to provide a series of hypotheses. This assessment feeds into the formulation, and this can be used to construct interventions to address a problem, encourage behaviours, improve well-being, and quality of life.

7.1 What is a neuropsychological formulation in the context of complex neuro-disability

The concept of formulation is understood and used in different ways by different professions working largely within mental health settings, and this can lead to some misunderstanding. Within clinical psychology and clinical neuropsychology, formulation is seen as a core skill and has been defined as 'a hypothesis about a person's difficulties, which links theory with practice and guides the intervention' (DCP, 2011). The Association of Clinical Psychologists further describe it as a 'Biopsychosocial formulation acknowledges a range of psychological, social, cultural and biological factors impacting on a person, and enables shared agreement about goals, intervention options and ways of managing challenges in creating change' (ACP, 2022). The psychological therapy or work that is then undertaken from this uses evidence-based therapeutic techniques (for example, using CBT for clinical depression), and the models underpinning these are often used to describe the formulation.

Formulations are often cocreated in a collaborative way with the person. Whilst this makes sense in the field of mental health, it is not feasible in the field of complex neuro-disability. When a patient has significantly altered cognitive and/or behavioural function, we also have to question whether we are dealing with the same problem as might be seen in a mental health setting. For example, we may observe that a person appears sad and is doing less than they were previously. Within a mental health setting, we might then make assumptions and generate hypotheses about mood and our formulation, goals and therapeutic actions are likely to be informed by our therapeutic skills/preferences. For example, if we prefer to work within a CBT approach, we might consider the difficulties in the context of how a person's behaviour is affected by their thinking. We can discuss this model with the person, reach some agreement about what is happening and then apply CBT techniques to support them to learn how to make changes in thinking patterns which result in an improvement in mood (e.g. explaining a list of common errors in thinking, exploring which might be relevant to them, getting them to spot these and then to challenge them and so on). For someone with complex neuro-disability, we may start with the same observations, they appear sad and they are not doing as much, but does this mean the same thing for this person and can we conclude that they too are depressed? There are a number of other considerations that might arise including:

- How does physical disability, pain, or medical illness impact on the person's activity levels?

- What is the impact of primary brain damage versus secondary reaction to changes in life on mood?
- How does cognitive impairment impact the person's experience of the world and hence on mood?
- How does cognitive impairment impact the person's ability to make use of talking therapies?
- How do cognitive and/or behavioural changes such as lack of insight, reduced initiation, or perseveration impact the presentation and/or the person's ability to engage in the possible therapies that might be offered?
- How might a life altering injury be understood by the person and impact on them?
- How might one or more of these factors impact on the person's ability to engage in the process of reaching a shared formulation?

However if, as we have seen above, the person's presentation is not sensibly described by a therapeutic model derived within a mental health setting, then it is not helpful to try to construct a formulation using that model. One must then question what other options are available. A very commonly used approach is a list approach to formulation. This is normally taught as the 5Ps approach described by MacNeil (2012), although different versions of this approach may have additional Ps! It seeks to address clinical questions of why is this person presenting in this way at this time, what keeps this problem in their life and what helps? The 5 Ps consist of 1) the presenting problem, 2) the predisposing factors, 3) the precipitating factors, 4) the perpetuating factors, and 5) the protective factors. The idea is that consideration of these five factors enables the clinician to take a systematic and holistic approach to formulating a person's problems. The formulation can then be used to build a rehabilitation programme with helpful and relevant interventions. However, it could be argued that this approach, though certainly helpful in terms of considering relevant areas and providing a systematic approach, does not enable one to properly integrate all the different threads, but rather lists matters in an additive way. It does not properly consider the dynamic relationship between cognition, behaviour, and emotion in detail, and specifically, does not consider the personal meaning of these different threads. Kinderman et al. (2008) comment on how the impact of difficult circumstances or events is mediated through the meaning that they hold for an individual, and following this, the DCP guidelines state that personal meaning is the integrating factor in a psychological formulation.

More recently, Thrower et al. (2024) set out to develop a consensus on the essential components of a formulation with the aim of informing training of clinical psychologists and updating best practice guidelines. They concluded that there was agreement that formulation should be client-led and incorporate strengths and sociocultural factors. However, looking at the consensus on both the essential components and processes in formulation, there are certainly difficulties in applying this to complex neuro-disability. In particular, although developing a shared formulation with family and other team members may be possible, it will usually not be possible to develop a shared formulation with the patient themselves.

It is also notable that the consensus statements agreed formulations were problem-focused. The emphasis of formulations is different in complex neuro-disability. It shifts the goalposts of formulation from 'what do we see and how does this explain the problem we are trying to solve?' to 'what do we see and how can we use this in any way to improve a person's quality of life?'. You will notice that the nature of this shift in focus also enables the idea of an iterative process – a need for developing and testing hypotheses in the formulation and then updating and refining the formulation as new information is reached.

For people who have suffered the most severe and catastrophic brain injuries and who now live with complex neuro-disability across multiple domains, formulation using the biopsychosocial model is helpful because it recognises the complex interaction between biological, psychological, behavioural, and social factors impacting on a person following such a devastating injury and provides a framework from which to consider rehabilitation in a more holistic way. A specific attempt to draw together the biopsychological and the ecological factors that need to be considered in the context of neurorehabilitation has been designed and described as a Holistic Neuropsychological Formulation Framework (Evans, Fish, Winegardner, Betteridge Sunak, Limond, Jim & Watson, personal communication based on a previous version by Evans 2006, as cited in Wilson et al., 2009; Figure 7.1). This approach to formulation makes clear factors relevant to who the person has been prior to their injury, and the values and beliefs that are idiosyncratic to that person, the ecological context, whilst making overt how the neurological injury is impacting on the various cognitive, communicative, physical, sensory, emotional, and behavioural functions. This approach may help derive a deeper, more meaningful, and personalised formulation and enables goal-setting congruent with the person's identity.

Although this approach to formulation can look complicated at first glance, within complex and severe brain injury, actually filling in the boxes can be even more complicated and potentially problematic. For example, there may be big question marks in the cognition box and the emotion and mood box, and the physical box may be a moving target with medical changes occurring rapidly. The emphasis of the different aspects of this model of formulation tend to be different for complex neuro-disability than for people with less severe brain injuries. Firstly, the extent of the biological injuries is greater and, as has been seen in earlier chapters, the consequence of this for rehabilitation is not simply one of intensity but rather successful rehabilitation shifts the goalposts of what the team is aiming to achieve. We are looking for 'ability', not trying to fix 'disability'. Secondly, the psychological and behavioural context is also different. Questions about the applicability of many of the psychological concepts that we work with in the rehabilitation of people with less severe brain injuries arise because of the extent of global cognitive

Developmental history and premorbid function ('Early Life')

Consider any factors relevant to aid understanding and characterisation of current functioning

Pre- and perinatal factors, developmental milestones, early learning environment, developmental adversity, neurodevelopmental disorders, education and attainment, social and emotional development, vocational history, premorbid roles, premorbid organisational systems and coping styles.

Psychosocial Context (Family & Social)

Nature and culture of the systems relevant to the person (pre and post injury info can be included)

Family (e.g. structure, identity, mottos)
Social situation and networks
Wider living environment
Educational and/or work environments
Culture, religion and community
Relevant supports and teams involved

Person

Identifying information
Name, age, gender

Neurological Condition ('Brain Stuff')

Relevant medical context
Diagnoses, dates, regions affected, severity, course, treatments +/- medications, outstanding questions

Identity ('Who I am')

Provide snapshot characterising what's most important to the person (pre and post, capturing important changes)

Subjective sense of self/self-representation
Values
Aspirations and expectations
Beliefs in relation to help, health, disability

Emotion and Mood

Adjustment (e.g. to injury/condition and to disability)
Mood
Anxiety
Anger
Emotion regulation (link to cog)
Beliefs about emotion
Coping style
Impact/interaction with premorbid mental health

Communication

Motor components
Cognitive components
Pure linguistic components
Expressive and receptive
Personal style
Variation across contexts

Behaviour of concern

Describe and use arrows
Can use separate box or locate in cog/comm/mood/physical according to case

Goals

Provide narrative ('headline message') to orient to rehab.
- Anchor goals in identity
- Highlight discrepancies if relevant
- GAS/SMART according to context

Cognition ('Thinking skills')

Characterise cognitive profile focussing on main areas of difficulty and strength. Use data from tests, observation, self and other report

Core domains:
Intellect
Attention
Speed of Processing
Executive
Memory

Supplementary domains:
Perceptual functions (link: sensory)
Social cognitive abilities
Calculation
Language

Participation & Functional Consequences ('Everyday consequences')

Describe impact on day to day tasks across a range of situations that are important to the person, and level of support needed.

ADLs, relationships, driving, community access, engagement with hobbies and interests, volunteering, work/education

Physical

Sensory and perceptual (vision, hearing, touch, taste, smell, proprioception, vestibular)
Motor
Endocrine
Issues commonly considered physical (sleep, fatigue, pain)
Other health conditions not actively contributing to neuro issues

Highlight box

Use to emphasise/illustrate interactive concepts or maintenance cycles

Loss
Insight/awareness

Template produced by: Jon Evans, Jess Fish, Jill Winegardner, Silke Betteridge, Sanjay Sunak, Jenny Limond, Jimmy Jim & Suzanne Watson

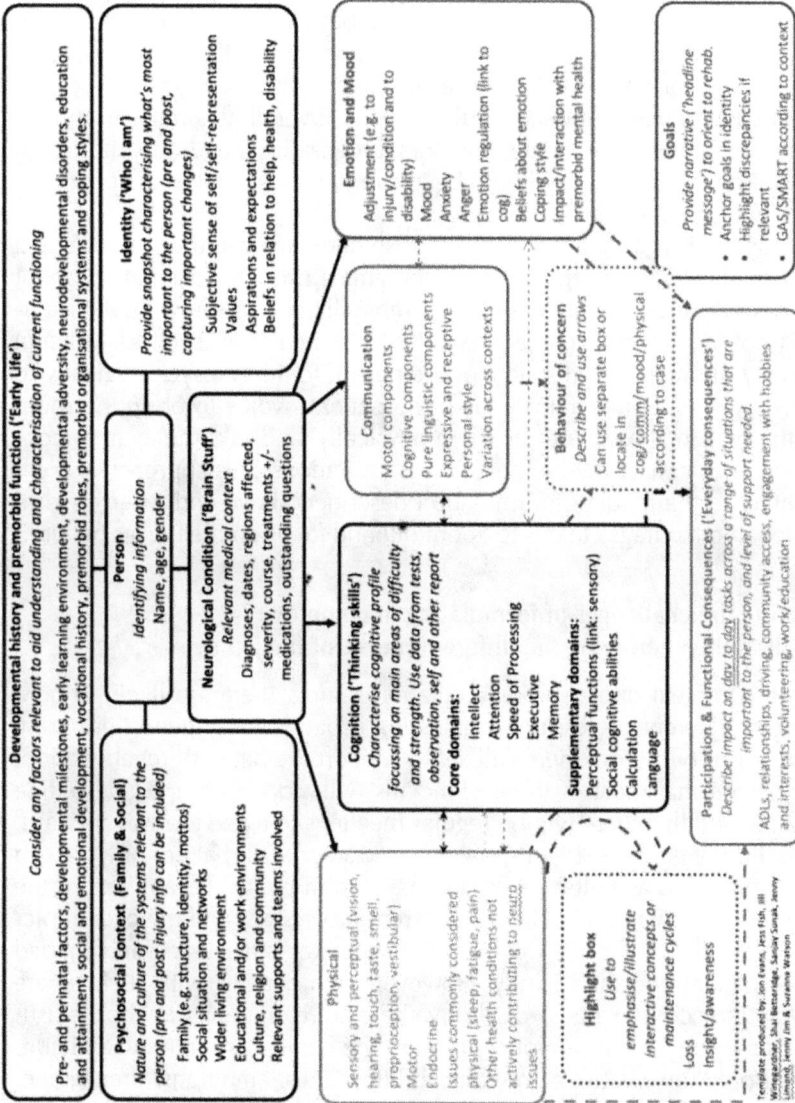

Figure 7.1 Holistic neuropsychological formulation framework (Evans, Fish, Winegardner, Betteridge Sunak, Limond, Jim & Watson, personal communication based on a previous version by Evans 2006, as cited in Wilson et al., 2009).

impairments in complex neuro-disability. Thirdly, the social factors influence matters in a different way. For example, changes in relationships or socio-economic matters are likely to be of much greater concern to relatives than those with complex neuro-disability who are very unlikely to be cognisant of them. Finally, preinjury characteristics may be far less important to the person in the context of so much global impairment but are just as important, if not more so, to their relatives. It should be remembered that the task is not to be able to fill information in all of these boxes, but rather to use the information you have to better understand the patient. Overall, this model can provide a useful guide to the range of factors to consider in neuropsychological rehabilitation, but clinicians should be aware of the challenges of applying it too rigidly to this complex patient group.

As described in Chapter 3, the use of spidergrams captures the values a person holds and their aspirations. Spidergrams provide information about a person's priorities and preferences for rehabilitation, even when the aspiration is not viewed by clinicians as able to be achieved (such as walking) which may allow time and space for the person to adjust psychologically to the new realities. Spidergrams enable the patient's voice to be in the room when the person is unable to be there physically, and asks the team to consider how they can help with the person's aspirations. This approach is complementary to the model of formulation described above and when used in conjunction encourages teams to zoom out and focus on the bigger picture.

7.2 Facing the challenges of formulating in complex neuro-disability: gathering the different pieces of the jigsaw

Within the context of a neurorehabilitation setting, there are likely to be a number of different professionals assessing a patient and then considering what they can offer from their skill set to support the patient's rehabilitation. It is expected that most of these clinicians will work within a goal-setting framework and that there will be regular meetings to agree the way forward, prioritisation of goals or streams to work, and so on. This pattern of work can be conceptualised as putting a jigsaw together. In typical rehabilitation, the different pieces are provided by the different professions and the overall picture, and the picture on the jigsaw box if you like, is discussed and shaped with the patient and their family. However, with patients with such severe and profound complex neuro-disability, the picture on the jigsaw box is usually missing. The patient cannot contribute. The family have in mind a picture derived from their relative's previous abilities, likes, ambitions, dreams etc, and the professionals are trying to build a picture without all the pieces and where there are no certainties – a jigsaw with no edge pieces and a lot of sky. In the absence of being able to conduct an assessment and hold all the pieces of the jigsaw in mind to then try to formulate with, the first step in complex neuro-disability is to collect as many of the pieces of the jigsaw as we are able to. To use the scientist–practitioner approach to test pieces and see if they are relevant. The next step is to consider whether we have any clues to what the overall picture on the box is, or even a part of the picture.

Professionals who are new to this work often feel very deskilled, and there is a tendency to fall back to focusing on identifying problems and trying to solve these. Clinicians describe a pressure or expectation that they should work on fixing things rather than managing the difficulties, and discussion of managing the difficulties is often seen as either giving up on the patient or alternatively it is taken as an indication that a rehabilitation setting is not appropriate. Adopting the stance of identifying a problem and trying to fix it allows the clinician to focus once more on a task that they can undertake with a patient and provides a sense of active engagement with the patient which is reinforcing in the short-term. Yet just doing something is often not helpful because taking this approach with someone whose behavioural repertoire is very limited frequently results in assumptions being made, frustration for staff and family, and a further sense of deskilling.

The other factor to consider is that in the context of brain injury, there may be more pieces in this jigsaw that you have not yet been able to obtain, or may never obtain. The team will be considering physical, task-orientated, sensory, medical, nutritional, pain, medication and its side-effects, sleep–wake cycles and fatigue management, and so on, in addition to cognitive, behavioural and emotional factors for a patient and their family, overall well-being for all, possible onward placement needs and adjustments to this and financial stresses on the patient or family. Although clinical psychologists and other professions are used to encountering a mix of these difficulties in many patient groups, it is arguable that with this group of patients who have experienced such a severe brain injury, they are often needing to consider many more, if not all of them, for the person. It goes without saying that these factors are not mutually exclusive but rather they impact each other and an additional goal of any rehabilitation programme will be to try to reach some sort of dynamic balance where the patient is enabled to experience the greatest engagement with their environment, social and physical, and the greatest sense of well-being and quality of life.

Formulating in this context requires a transdisciplinary approach (see Chapter 11). Formulation, goals, and tasks are made together by the different professions involved, and where possible the patient and their family team, with the focus of the programme developed from the patient needs rather than being profession-specific. Once this formulation is made and there is a shared understanding of what the programme is aiming to achieve, how these matters might be addressed and who/which skills are best placed to achieve this can be organised. Formulations themselves are dynamic and not static. They need to be progressively refined and regularly updated as new data, and information is available and as the person themselves changes.

The results of assessments from the different professionals provide many of the pieces of the jigsaw, but the nature of these pieces can be very different. Some assessments may provide a clear starting point for an intervention. For example, weight, height, blood test results, and activity levels may provide a clear guide for a skilled dietitian to work out the starting point of a nutrition regime for someone who is PEG fed, and a good nutritional regime is clearly the foundation of all other aspects of rehabilitation. However, observation of behaviour may lead to a series of hypotheses about the purpose of that behaviour, and these will require testing and refinement. Working with people who have limited movement and no language is likely to complicate this process further. It is also the case that in general terms, the rate of change with this group of patients is extremely slow. In this context, the sense of pressure to do something that comes from family and funders alike can result in members of the team falling into the trap of making assumptions about what a behaviour may mean, rather than allowing the time and space to go through the necessary process of developing and testing hypotheses.

Neuropsychologists are often dealing directly with areas where there is no immediate answer to questions and working out what may be going on takes a significant amount of time. There is inevitably a period of uncertainty, and this can be both frustrating and distressing for family members. Family, with their background knowledge of a patient's pre-brain injury personality and behaviour pattern, are very likely to interpret behaviours and make assumptions about what these may demonstrate. The problem is that assumptions made on the basis of premorbid characteristics or skills may or may not be accurate. However, hearing that message from a professional who has no prior knowledge of their loved one can be interpreted as arrogant and presumptuous. This is not a good way to set up rapport with a patient's family.

In contrast with the family, therapists start from what they observe in the person in front of them and what is happening now. They have no pre-existing knowledge of that person and their individuality. In situations where things do not change fast, the professionals working with the patient base their opinion and plan their programme largely based on their knowledge of what is usual and what the general trends are for this group of patients. Their opinion, at least initially, cannot be based on the individual patient themselves. In constructing the picture then we have family and friends of the injured person basing their view on their past knowledge of the person and their hopes and dreams for the future (getting back what has been lost). By contrast, the professional team is basing their opinion on what they see before them, and their knowledge of the general pattern of recovery of people injured in this way (developing only what might be possible). There is potential for conflict in building an individualised rehabilitation programme here because the foundations of these opinions are different, and although one might usually expect the patient's goals and views to provide the unifying material, in this patient group that is often not possible. The skill of neuropsychological formulation here is to see both approaches and to be able to hold both and meld them so that rather than a conflict, there is a richer picture to work from. Sometimes it is necessary to hold two pictures, perhaps because two hypotheses are being tested or perhaps because each represents a different part of a larger picture.

It is often the case that the greater the complexity of a patient's situation, the larger the number of professionals involved. Each profession is contributing to the picture and each profession has an important contribution to make, but how these contributions are linked and how to prioritise these needs consideration. Referring back to the jigsaw analogy, we see that the greater the number of professionals involved, the more pieces we are trying to fit together. It is clear which way up some of these pieces should go but how other pieces fit, their orientation, and which part of the puzzle they belong to, may require trial and error across the whole programme. This demonstrates the need for collaboration across the whole professional team and family, friends, and other key figures in a patient's life. It is not uncommon to hear families reflect that 'no one knows' what may be possible or 'how brains really work'. This collaboration is being attempted in often deeply distressing circumstances for the family and with competing time pressures for the practitioners, and this emotion needs to be contained when trying to develop a formulation and then move forward from formulation to rehabilitation plan. This is an important role for the neuropsychologist.

Psychologists are skilled at balancing and managing contributions of groups of people, as well as eliciting views of others, managing conflicting views and emotional distress, and summarising and integrating ideas. In meetings where formulation and rehabilitation programmes are discussed, particularly if the person is not present, then the neuropsychologist should use their person-centred skills to ensure that the person is held at the centre of all discussions, and that their interests, beliefs, and values are represented. As a profession, we are skilled at managing the strong emotions that are likely to arise in discussions regarding formulation and in asking what may be challenging questions, either of family or our colleagues. We are also able to identify and manage the personal views and biases of the people attending any meeting and be aware of working sensitively with issues of diversity and cultural needs. It is often the case that the less able a patient is to interact in any sense, the stronger the expression of personal views becomes in such meetings and the higher the emotional temperature can become if there is debate or disagreement. Being aware of this and actively managing it is something that the neuropsychologist should ensure is addressed in formulating as a team.

In order to play the sort of role described above, the psychologist must have face validity in the team. It is important that neuropsychologists are integrated and part of the wider team and not separated both geographically and in the team culture (behind a desk with tests on). Once one has demonstrated an ability to value contributions from across the team and synthesise them and draw a team formulation together, the team will recognise and respect this contribution that psychologists can make. There can be a sense of a power battle in teams, and it can be easy to find oneself sucked into such battles, even inadvertently. It is helpful to keep in mind that respect is very different from power and very much more helpful in this scenario. Once respect has been gained, it becomes self-perpetuating.

If a team is going to build a formulation together, then the jigsaw pieces they use must be from the same box. The language that is used by members of the team must be shared. For example, words such as significant, reliable, aware, behavioural, functional, aggression, and agitation are used in different ways by different people in different settings. Some people use aggression and agitation interchangeably and some see agitation as a lesser form of aggression. If people are trying to agree on a formulation but using the same words to mean different things, then any sharing will be weak at best and probably highly frustrating for both the patient and the team. We do not necessarily question whether we are applying the same meaning to words or not in case reviews. It is a good idea, particularly where there is some friction in the discussions, to check and ensure that we are applying the same meanings. This is also true when working with families, it is common to hear discussions that use clinical jargon and alienate people (such as 'upper limbs' instead of 'arms').

7.3 Using the formulation to plan the rehabilitation programme: putting the jigsaw together

The most successful neurorehabilitation programmes with this group of patients require not only teamwork but a shared formulation by the team, and the clinical neuropsychologist has a key role to play in bringing about a shared formulation. It is worth considering how one can bring about a truly shared formulation where there is a real sense that the team shares not only a description of the presentation but also understands and agrees the tasks/ interventions that are planned and the order and prioritisation of these. There is something very powerful about working within a team where it is possible to achieve this. It requires significant trust between team members and the ability to consider things from a transdisciplinary perspective. The neuropsychologist has a key role to play in bringing this about for a number of reasons.

Inevitably with this group of patients, much of the work undertaken is focused on the body, the person's physical needs, rather than on the person. By contrast as psychologists, it is our role to focus on the person, and it is our skill to bring the person back into the room during team discussions. This may or may not be literally. Within neurorehabilitation, there is an expectation that the person receiving the rehabilitation should be part of planning and goal-setting meetings and should be included in discussions about the development of their rehabilitation programme and where they are able to engage with such a meeting this is important. However, having the person (literally in body) in the room with all the professionals may not be the best way of including the patient or enabling them to engage with the planning of rehabilitation. It is clear that some patients cannot be involved at any level, for example those in VS, but there are many patients whose abilities and resilience levels leave them in a grey area, where careful consideration of the purpose and the pros and cons of bringing them into a large meeting should be carefully considered. Involving a person in the development of their rehabilitation, where that is possible, is a fundamental principle of person-centred rehabilitation, but having them in a meeting they are unable to participate in might be considered tokenistic at best and potentially harmful at worst. It is necessary to consider issues around their capacity, sharing information, and not causing undue distress. Consideration must be given to how they are able to contribute to the meeting, how long they can concentrate, their communication abilities (receptively and expressively), what ability they have to cope with the attentional switching demands between so many participants, the inclusivity of language, their stage of self-awareness and insight into their condition and needs, their ability to hold information in mind, their ability to emotionally regulate when the focus is on difficult topics etc. Whether the person is present or not, how their views and values are reflected in the planning and prioritisation of a rehabilitation programme is key.

Whatever the decision is about whether and how a person can be involved in the development of a formulation, it is important to be very transparent about what the patient's involvement is and for whom. For some patients being able to identify their priorities is possible but for others, being present in the meeting may mean being present in the minds of the professionals as a person, not a patient. This recognition of the person prior to the injury is often commented on by staff who see photographs of the person prior to their injury. This can have a very moving impact on the member of staff, and it is always worth reflecting on this when we are formulating for a person, and when considering our own responses to that person. Keeping them in mind as what is sometimes described by relatives as the 'whole person' as opposed to the 'broken' one they are currently trying to mend.

Psychologists have strong skills in synthesising information. We are taught analytical skills, how to consider all information in the round and to check for validity and reliability before drawing conclusions. We are taught on the one hand to be curious about all aspects of a picture and on the other to be suspicious and to check what information is actually telling us (see Chapters 4 and 5 on cognition and behaviour). We're good at critical appraisal, taking the information and pulling it together, seeing beyond the individual pieces, looking for the bigger picture, pulling out from the detail to see the whole. Many different professionals come with a view of the part of the picture that they are involved in building but may not know how this might fit with the bigger overall picture. This is one area in which clinical neuropsychologists have strong skills, being able to see the bigger picture and sharing an understanding that the whole is more than the sum of its parts.

The first part of the task in building a shared formulation is to highlight what the team does know and what it does not know and where the team agrees on matters or disagrees. Following this, an agreement of what the team needs to do next can be brought out. Within the context of team discussions, neuropsychologists might not simply accept what others have concluded. We question what they have found, how that might link to the conclusion they have drawn, and what the method they used to gather and assess the data was. In doing this, we are not trying to undermine our colleagues' skills but rather bringing our specialist knowledge and experience to evaluate the quality of the evidence and/or whether the piece does show what the practitioner says it does.

7.4 Good practice tips

- Feeling deskilled is normal and it is okay, everyone working in this area experiences this.
- You cannot synthesise information until you've actually heard the information. Your voice being silent for periods of time in a case review is okay.
- Your job is to keep the big picture in mind (e.g. discharge planning – where are they going, what needs to happen first?)
- Your job is to be able to sit with uncertainty (what are the uncertainties and what are we going to do to achieve certainty?).
- There is always too much information. You have to filter to work out the critical pieces.
- Because we are principally involved in cognition, emotion, and behaviour, we are paying attention to details other people might have missed – e.g. 'are you sure they could see it? It sounds like all those sessions happened on their left hand side'
- Look out for assumptions and interrogate them. For example, just because everyone says 'it's this' we should not simply accept it. We need to question clinical reasoning to make it more robust, 'are you sure it couldn't be this?' or 'how did you rule out that?'
- Actively draw on your knowledge of neuroanatomy, cognitive functioning and behavioural principles. This is certainly a complex field and can feel like guesswork to start with, but it's not unknowable.
- Indulge your intellectual curiosity in the need for detective work. It is always interesting and novel and intellectually rewarding to work with this client group.
- Foster your tolerance for uncertainty. It is possible to move forward in what might feel like chaos.
- Remember that you can do something that contributes to a patient's quality of life after something so devastating has happened.
- Keeping a focus on what we should do, not what we can do. We are looking at quality of life for a person whose whole way of life and sense of self has been blown apart, not seeing how far we can pursue possibly miniscule gains.
- Always keep in mind when it is time to stop. Seeing this is harder if you are trying to fix things.

7.5 Dealing with clinical challenges in complex formulation

The majority of clinical neuropsychologists do not come across this group of clients on a regular basis and so are unlikely to have a great deal of experience in working with them. Furthermore, the tools and models that a neuropsychologist may fall back on when meeting a new client are not always useful with this group of people. The result, as mentioned earlier in this chapter, is that the neuropsychologist may feel quite deskilled when assessing and formulating the needs of a patient. This is not only true for the neuropsychologist on a team but also for many other professionals whose skills are required in the development of a rehabilitation programme for the patient. The box highlights some of the challenges that teams should be aware of.

Clinical challenges in complex case formulation

- When people feel deskilled, they can become anxious about the value they bring to thinking about a formulation. When anxious they are more likely to preciously guard their piece in the jigsaw and to highlight its value. They become less able to step back from that and to find or to view the bigger picture.
- Different roles also bring different levels of certainty. Some roles are more task-based and have greater predictability or routine than others. Those members of the team who deal with the less predictable or routine matters sometimes feel a sense of frustration from colleagues that they are not fixing the problems that stand in the way of further progress. For example, many neuropsychologists will have heard comments such as 'Rehabilitation can't start until you have sorted the behaviour', with little understanding that fixing the behaviour is a very significant part of rehabilitation.
- Team members will be working at different speeds depending on the complexity of their role and the certainty or task-based nature of their role. Managing priorities and pressures from funders can be difficult to do in this context.
- The government paperwork, such as the Decision Support Tool for NHS Continuing Healthcare, upon which a person's funding depends, is arguably more difficult to fill out for sections that psychologists might see as their particular area of expertise, psychological and emotional, cognition, and behaviour. This is in part because the levelling of these aspects of care does demand a level of interpretation rather than a tangible measure. It is arguable that the levels set out for cognition do not capture many of the most challenging aspects of cognitive deficit following a brain injury, where care is likely to be needed but difficult to deliver well. These areas are also areas where

---

everyone feels they have an equal say. It is often those patients that sit at the boundaries between levels when everyone involved is likely to offer their opinion most vociferously, and it can be harder for the expert in the area to make their voice heard. Whereas assessors are likely to defer to a specialist medical or physiotherapy opinion but not necessarily to one regarding emotion or behaviour (and sometimes cognition) presented by a neuropsychologist.

- What to do about issues of mental capacity. In most settings, rehabilitation is done with consent, where you explain your assessment and intervention plan and the patient either gives informed consent or refuses. In our setting, the patient will either lack the capacity to consent to treatment, and intervention will be in their best interests, or they may have capacity for some decisions but not others. Progress is not linear with this group of patients, and it is necessary to be aware of change and to be responsive to the management of changes and/or possible fluctuations in capacity to make different decisions regarding aspects of rehabilitation.
- Risk aversion can have a very negative impact on planning or delivering aspects of rehabilitation. Staff and/or the organisation fear reputation damage, being struck-off or performance management where risks are taken on behalf of patient's who lack capacity to consent to a particular programme. Be clear on the value and rights of positive risk-taking.
- The emphasis in note writing shifts from a description of what the member of staff has done that can be used as a guide either for themselves or for another practitioner to carry on with the work, and becomes more about defensive practice, proving that the practitioner has done what they are 'supposed to do'.

7.6 In summary: what does a good formulation look like?

It will be clear from this chapter that describing a 'good' formulation is not a straightforward task! To use our jigsaw analogy, it is a bit like the satisfaction a group of people feel on completing a 10,000-piece abstract jigsaw puzzle from a starting point where there was no picture to guide them, they couldn't find most of the pieces, and everyone was arguing about where to start. It is not even as simple as drawing an example picture of a completed puzzle, or giving a hypothetical set of completed boxes using the Evans model cited earlier. This is because the formulation is not just the picture at the end, it is the process of steps which transformed each earlier attempt at the puzzle into the end-product. This combination of product and process is what makes it difficult to provide a tangible illustration. Also, the use of the jigsaw puzzle analogy should not be interpreted as meaning that the perfect picture will have been fully completed by the end of this phase of rehabilitation. As will be clear, it is highly unlikely that the people with complex neuro-disability and their families will perceive this to be the case. However, agreeing on when there is a sufficiently clear picture to stop is an important part of a good process. In summary, here is a list of factors that contribute to a 'good' formulation:

- It is written within a clear context of the aims of rehabilitation and what is or would be most important to the person themselves
- It includes a clear understanding of their areas of difficulty and how these interact with each other. This understanding builds over time. The formulation is a process not a static model.
- At each stage, the process of prioritising and allocating interventions is clear, and there are opportunities to resolve conflicts.
- The person is kept at the centre of building this understanding and prioritising interventions. This can be figuratively for those who cannot voice their opinions, or literally for those people who can contribute, but with careful thought given to how to optimise their involvement.
- The family are part of the team and collaborate with building the formulation and identifying priorities.
- There is a clear understanding of when the picture is complete enough to stop, so that the person can be supported to move on. When the process has worked well there is a shared satisfaction amongst the person, their family, and the clinical team that their needs were understood, and they are ready for the next step in their rehabilitation journey.

References

Association of Clinical Psychologists. (2022). *Team Formulation: Key Considerations in Mental Health Services*. Association of Clinical Psychologists

Division of Clinical Psychology. (2011). *Good Practice Guidelines on the Use of Psychological Formulation*. British Psychological Society.

Kinderman, P., Sellwood, W., & Tai, S. (2008). Policy implications of a psychological model of mental disorder. *Journal of Mental Health*, *17*(1), 93–103.

MacNeil, C. A., Hasty, M. K., Conus, P., & Berk, M. (2012). Is diagnosis enough to guide interventions in mental health? Using case formulation in clinical practice. *BMC Medicine*, *10*, 111. https://Doi.org/10.1186/1741-7015-10-111

Thrower, N. E., Bucci, S., Morris, L., & Berry, K. (2024). The key components of a clinical psychology formulation: A consensus study. *The British Journal of Clinical Psychology*, *63*, 2, 213–226. https://DOI.org/10.1111/bjc.12455

Wilson, B. A. (2017). The development of neuropsychological rehabilitation: An historical examination of theoretical and practical issues pp 6–17. In B. A. Wilson, J. Winegardner, C. M. van Heugten, & T. Ownsworth (Eds.) *Neuropsychological Rehabilitation: The International Handbook*. Routledge.

Wilson, B.A, Gracey, F., Evans, J. J., & Bateman, A. (Eds) (2009). *Neuropsychological Rehabilitation: Theory, Models, Therapy and Outcomes*. Cambridge University Press. ISBN 9780521841498.

8 Working with people with prolonged disorders of consciousness

8.1 Definitions

Disorders of consciousness (DOC) occur when brain injury is so severe that the person shows limited or no evidence of awareness at any time. A 'prolonged' disorder of consciousness (PDOC) is defined as a disorder of consciousness lasting longer than 28 days (RCP, 2020; Giacino et al., 2018). Such disorders can occur following any type of sudden onset acquired brain injury, including traumatic brain injury, stroke, and hypoxic injuries (Royal College of Physicians (RCP, 2020). It is important to know the aetiology of the injury when determining prognosis for recovery over time, as discussed later in this chapter. PDOC-like states can also occur in late-stage progressive illnesses such as dementia, when they are termed a 'terminal disorder of consciousness (TDOC), although this chapter will focus on those with ABI in line with professional practice guidelines (RCP, 2020). Even defining terms such as 'consciousness' and 'awareness' is challenging as there is no single medical investigation that can determine these with certainty; assessment therefore depends on inferring consciousness from behaviour or its absence.

Disorders of consciousness are rare, with incidence estimated to be around 2.6 per 100,000 people per year, and prevalence estimated to be around 2-5 per 100,000 people, with some variation between countries (Wade, 2018). The principal professional practice guidelines relating to PDOC in the UK are those written by the Royal College of Physicians, the most recent iteration of which, at the time of writing, was the revision published in 2020 (RCP, 2020). The RCP (2020) guidelines delineate DOC into coma, vegetative state (VS) and minimally conscious state (MCS) as described in the following box:

DOI: 10.4324/9781032665986-8

Definitions of disorders of consciousness

Condition	Definition	Description
Coma	Absent wakefulness and absent awareness	A state of unrousable unresponsiveness, lasting more than 6 hours in which a person: • is unconscious with closed eyes and cannot be awakened • fails to respond normally to painful stimuli, light or sound • lacks a normal sleep–wake cycle • does not initiate voluntary actions.
Vegetative state (VS)	Wakefulness with absent awareness	A state of wakefulness without awareness in which there is preserved capacity for spontaneous or stimulus-induced arousal – evidenced by sleep–wake cycles and a range of reflexive and spontaneous behaviours. VS is characterised by absence of behavioural evidence for self or environmental awareness.
Minimally conscious state (MCS)	Wakefulness with minimal awareness	A state of severely altered consciousness in which minimal but clearly discernible behavioural evidence of self or environmental awareness is demonstrated MCS is characterised by inconsistent, but reproducible, responses above the level of spontaneous or reflexive behaviour, which indicate some degree of interaction with their surroundings

Although the main distinction made between coma and VS in the table is around the presence or absence of wakefulness, it is important to highlight that this is not just about the presence/absence of eye-opening. Unlike patients in coma, those in VS can show a wide range of behaviours. These can include gross motor behaviours such as limb or head movements, finer motor behaviours such as finger movements, eyebrow raises or tongue or lip movements, and behaviours which are usually associated with emotional experiences such as smiling and grimacing. These behaviours are compatible with the diagnosis of VS provided they occur spontaneously or as reflexive responses rather than as purposeful or environmentally contingent responses (RCP, 2020). However, the challenge for the clinician working with these patients is obvious – how can the clinician be certain about the intent or otherwise of a behaviour? Whilst specific methods of assessment are discussed in more detail in the second part of this chapter, the principles of objectivity versus subjectivity, careful structured observations, hypothesis testing, and caution in interpreting findings are key factors to hold in mind when working with this group of patients.

There are some variations in how terminology is used internationally. The most commonly used alternative to 'vegetative state' is 'unresponsive wakefulness syndrome' (UWS), a term coined by the European Task Force on DOC in response to concerns from both clinicians and the public about 'vegetative' potentially being misinterpreted as 'vegetable-like', and to a desire to emphasise the lack of responsiveness, which is observable, rather than lack of awareness, which can only be inferred (Laureys et al., 2010). American practice guidelines for DOC, which were updated in 2018 and reaffirmed in 2024, use both terms ('VS/UWS') throughout (Giacino et al., 2018).

As can be seen from the definitions above, the key difference between a diagnosis of VS versus MCS is that patients in MCS show evidence of some, albeit limited, awareness, as evidenced by inconsistent but reproducible behaviours that indicate some interaction with their surroundings (Giacino et al., 2002). An additional challenge with MCS is the relatively recent distinction between 'higher' level behavioural responses, giving rise to a diagnosis of 'MCS+', and 'lower' level behavioural responses which are associated with a diagnosis of 'MCS-' (Bruno et al., 2011). Behaviours that are compatible with a diagnosis of MCS- include visual tracking of objects, automatic localized behaviours such as pulling at a bed sheet, or emotional responses such as smiling or crying that are triggered by emotionally salient (not neutral) stimuli. Conversely, patients with a diagnosis of MCS+ are identified via communicative behaviours such as command following, intelligible vocalisations and/or some ability to communicate yes and no responses, albeit inconsistently (Bruno et al., 2011).

Historically, the distinction between VS and MCS held a particular significance in the UK because the diagnosis of VS was seen as pivotal when considering whether life-sustaining treatments might be discontinued due to the 'futility' of treatment; however, evolutions in case law towards a more general best interests approach under the Mental Capacity Act (2005), have influenced a shift away from strict diagnostic labels, towards a consideration of the culture, beliefs and values of the individual, and the likelihood of them regaining a quality of life that they would personally value (RCP, 2020). Issues around continuing or discontinuing life-sustaining treatment for people who lack capacity are discussed in more detail in Chapter 2 and later in this chapter, but the purpose of highlighting this here is that current UK guidelines outline that the distinction between VS/MCS– versus MCS+ is more significant for determining the prognosis for significant recovery than the previous focus on VS versus MCS (RCP, 2020).

Operational criteria for determining emergence from MCS were outlined when the diagnostic category of MCS was first proposed (Giacino et al., 2002) and consisted of the patient either being able to demonstrate reliable and consistent communication (defined as being able to accurately answer 6/6 closed situational questions on two consecutive occasions), and/or being able to demonstrate knowledge of objects (defined as being able to use two different objects appropriately on two consecutive occasions). These criteria still apply in the USA. However, they have been criticised for a range of reasons including the potential for patients to fail the tasks due to reasons such as aphasia, apraxia, or agnosia, rather than disordered consciousness (see Nakase-Richardson et al., 2008; Pundole & Crawford, 2018). The 2020 revision of the UK guidelines broadened the communication criteria to include biographical as well as situational questions and added an additional paradigm such that patients can be said to have emerged from PDOC if they are able to select the correct picture from a choice of two on 6/6 occasions in two consecutive sessions (RCP, 2020). The guideline authors acknowledged the likelihood of some clinicians disagreeing about these criteria, but argued in favour of a conservative approach in order to avoid the risk of patients who only narrowly meet thresholds for emergence potentially being denied access to the specialist-funded care they need. Debate around these issues has continued, and a survey of UK clinicians working in specialist rehabilitation centres showed that more than three quarters of them (78.6%) believed that they had worked with patients who had emerged from PDOC but were unable to demonstrate this using the current operational definitions (Pundole et al., 2021).

Whilst there may be some grey area between the distinctions between VS/MCS–, MCS–/MCS+, and MCS+/emergence, the need for a thorough assessment of the person who is hypothesised to be in PDOC is clear as any behaviours they can demonstrate, and any patterns of change in profile over time, form a vital part of the process of diagnosis, prognosis, and clinical management. In the early stages post-injury, there is a need to rule out any reversible causes of their reduced consciousness, optimise the patient's physical condition, meet their care needs across each 24-hour period (given their total dependence on others), and observe their behaviour for signs of awareness, communication and cognitive intent. Close team working is important, acknowledging that while each discipline brings its own areas of particular specialty, there are also areas of overlap between roles. For example, determining whether a tracheostomy can be weaned is likely to involve input from medical, physiotherapy, SLT, and nursing staff; carrying out assessments of awareness and responsiveness is likely to involve input from SLT, OT, and neuropsychology, in addition to discussing any informal observations reported by the wider team. Practice guidelines emphasise the need for a specialist team who have expertise in PDOC, with the UK guidelines outlining that key disciplines are *'physiotherapy, occupational therapy, speech and language therapy, neuropsychology, nursing, and rehabilitation medicine'* (RCP, 2020). The guidelines also contain definitions of the skills and experience needed for a clinician to be considered an 'Expert PDOC Physician' or 'Expert PDOC Assessor' (RCP, 2020, annex 2b). This need for team specialism is also a key recommendation in the American practice guidelines, which highlight a range of risks associated with providing non-specialist input, including higher risks of mortality, medical complications, misdiagnosis, and both under- and over-estimation of prognosis (Giacino et al., 2018). The need for this expertise is underlined by evidence that misdiagnosis occurs in around 30–40% of patients (see Schnakers et al., 2009; Wang et al., 2020).

When optimal care is provided, it is expected that patients who experience some organic neurological recovery will show a wider range of behaviour over time, potentially progressing from VS to MCS and then emerging from PDOC. However, it is also the case that the brain injury is so severe in a subset of these patients that they will never regain any functional communication or independence. The probability of emergence varies with aetiology, with ongoing change more likely following a TBI than a hypoxic injury as time goes on. This difference is reflected in UK guidelines via variability of the recommended timeframes by which a DOC can be labelled as 'chronic' or 'permanent'. The RCP (2020) suggests the term 'continuing' VS or MCS when the patient has been in the same state of disordered consciousness for 4 weeks or longer – although in clinical practice we find that 'PDOC' is the term generally used. Their recommended timeframes for considering a DOC to be 'chronic' are illustrated in the following table:

Diagnosis	Anoxic or metabolic injury	Traumatic brain injury
Chronic VS	> 3 months	> 1 year
Chronic MCS-	> 3 months	> 1 year
Chronic MCS+	> 9 months	> 18 months

Although the term 'permanent' VS or MCS has become less commonly used over time, the RCP guidelines suggest that it can be helpful in guiding expectations. These guidelines state that if any of the above chronic conditions have remained unchanged for 6 months, i.e. with no trajectory of change (as measured by the

Coma Recovery Scale-Revised (CRS-R)), then the condition can be said to be permanent (i.e. 'permanent VS', 'permanent MCS-', or 'permanent MCS+'). This state of permanence can only be diagnosed by an Expert PDOC Physician (RCP, 2020). It is acknowledged that 'permanent' in this case means 'highly improbable', and there are documented cases of late emergence (see Yelden et al, 2018; Illman & Crawford, 2018; Dhamapurkar et al., 2016), although the RCP guidelines emphasise that such cases are rare. There is nevertheless some evidence that patients who do show some recovery after being in PDOC following TBI can continue to make functional gains up to ten years post-injury (Hammond et al, 2019; Nakamura et al, 2023). In addition to the aetiology, time since injury, and any pattern of change in responsiveness, other factors which impact upon prognosis include age and medical stability (RCP, 2020).

8.2 Behavioural assessments of awareness

In the UK, professional practice guidelines recommend using data from both formal and informal behavioural methods to guide diagnosis. Although other diagnostic and prognostic techniques using methods such as EEG and functional imaging (fMRI/PET) have been documented in the research literature (and are mentioned briefly later in the chapter), these are not currently endorsed as necessary in clinical practice (RCP, 2020), although this stance has been criticised as risking missing people with so called 'covert consciousness' or 'cognitive motor dissociation' (Scolding et al., 2021). This section will first summarise the main formal measures used in the UK, and then consider how to carry out an informal but hypothesis-driven approach to assessment.

8.2.1 Formal tools for assessing awareness and responsiveness

The accepted international gold standard tool for assessing awareness and responsiveness is the Coma Recovery Scale – Revised (CRS-R; Giacino et al., 2004). Clinicians working with this patient group should be familiar with this measure and be able to administer it, particularly as UK guidelines state that if only one formal measurement tool for awareness is used, then it should be this one (RCP, 2020). The CRS-R consists of six hierarchical scales in which higher scores denote higher levels of behavioural responsiveness. The assessor starts each scale with the highest ability item, and if the patient is able to pass this item the scale is discontinued. If the patient fails the item, the assessor works their way down the scale until either a pass is achieved, or the patient fails to demonstrate even basic reflexive responses.

Advantages of the CRS-R include its universal use, its relatively short speed of administration, its usefulness in discriminating between VS and MCS (Giacino et al., 2004), and ability to provide more accurate diagnoses than clinical consensus for VS, MCS, and emergence (Schakers et al., 2009). From the perspective of our clinical practice, disadvantages include the linguistic and cognitive complexity of some of the instructions (e.g. asking the patient 'am I touching my ear right now?' whilst touching one's nose), and the need to start at the highest end of each scale given that our patients will invariably be more impaired than this. Attendance on a formal training programme for the CRS-R is useful but not required. We have found that errors in administration are easily made and strongly recommend practicing administration with a colleague experienced in its use, prior to carrying out CRS-R assessments with patients, and viewing training videos (e.g. we have produced such videos for in-house training in collaboration with SLT colleagues).

Other tools that are recommended for use in the UK include the Wessex Head Injury Matrix (WHIM; Shiel et al, 2000) and the Sensory Modality Assessment and Rehabilitation Technique (SMART; Gill-Thwaites & Munday 2004). The WHIM is a 62-item behavioural scale. Behaviours are ordered from most basic to most complex, and the clinician records the total number of behaviours observed, and the number associated with the 'highest' behaviour seen. Advantages of the WHIM include its ease of administration, which means that observations can be made in a range of settings and by a variety of people. For example, behaviours seen at rest can be compared and contrasted with behaviours seen during care tasks, therapy sessions or family interactions. Research has found the standing position is associated with more behaviours than in sitting or lying (Elliott et al., 2005; Wilson et al., 2013). Families can also be offered the opportunity to score a WHIM alongside a clinician as a way of fostering collaborative formulation and/or psychoeducation if interpretations of behaviour differ. Disadvantages include elements of subjectivity, and some caution is needed in interpretation of the two scores given that factors such as physical and sensory disabilities can impact the number of behaviours the patient can potentially exhibit, and the evidence that the hierarchical ordering of the scale may not map accurately onto the levels of awareness and responsiveness shown by patients (Turner-Stokes et al., 2015). Nevertheless, provided the clinician is aware of the pros and cons of this scale and is prepared to consider the findings within the context of a broader-based approach to assessment then the WHIM can form a valuable part of the process.

The SMART was designed as an in-depth assessment of behaviours seen in each different sensory domain, including taste, smell and touch as well as visual and auditory. Each domain is ordered hierarchically from least to most complex behaviours seen. Advantages of the SMART include its inclusion of domains in which patients who are blind and deaf may be able to demonstrate awareness, and the thorough descriptions of behaviours it generates. Disadvantages include the relatively lengthy time of administration, lack of discontinue criteria, and the number of sessions needed to generate a full report (ten sessions, each lasting up to 90 minutes, although more recent evidence suggests that 5-6 are sufficient (da Conceição Teixeira et al., 2021). In addition, the SMART can only be administered by those who have undertaken specific training. In our clinical experience, the strict manualised approach of SMART is less useful for clinical neuropsychologists than applying our scientist–practitioner principles to informal assessments (described briefly below). However, when a SMART has been carried out by another team member, the findings are valuable in developing the team formulation, alongside data from the CRS-R and/or WHIM, and any other measures of awareness and responsiveness which may have been used, such as the STAR (Sensory Tool to Assessment Responsiveness, Stokes et al., 2018) and the MATADOC (Music Therapy Tool to Assess DOC, Magee et al., 2014).

We have found that it is helpful to present the obtained results of these measures to illustrate whether or not there is a true trajectory of change in a patient's presentation or not over time. It can be useful for staff, funders, and families to have a visual graph showing the total score possible (make sure you graph so the Y axis has the total score possible) and the obtained scores plotted over time (the X axis). It can be helpful to add colour blocks to show where people typically score in VS as opposed to MCS– and MCS+, so that the obtained score is contextualised. We have worked with people in PDOC over many years, and having scores plotted from the acute hospital, the post-acute and long-term care assessments can be powerful. We also have a preference to include the impact of any intervention attempts on the graph for example if Zolpidem or Amantadine medications are trialled as potential treatments for level of awareness (by adding the time point on the X axis showing this).

8.2.2 Informal approaches to assessing awareness and responsiveness

The importance of using both formal validated tools in combination with clinical examinations and informal observations is highlighted in professional practice guidelines (RCP, 2020). Broader medical and other physical examinations are considered such as ruling out other potential medical reasons for the patient's presentation and testing the primary sensory (such as Brainstem Auditory Evoked Potentials (BAEPs) and Flash Visual Evoked Potentials (VEPs)) and motor pathways (such as Somatosensory Evoked Potentials (SSEP)). Evoked potential studies measure electrical activity in the brain in response to stimulation of sight, sound, or touch. For example, if a person is not observed to have any functional vision, such as not consistently showing a startle or attending to visual stimuli, then an assessment of whether the optic nerve pathway is intact (VEP) can be helpful in determining if this is in all probability due to the extensive damage to brain regions normally devoted to understanding the environment visually. It is assumed that such findings will be discussed in team case review meetings and/or available in shared records as part of the team approach.

Prior to each assessment of awareness, it is important that you observe the patient for 5–10 minutes without any stimulation in order to identify spontaneous behaviours. This is to ensure these are not be misinterpreted as voluntary and purposeful responses to stimulation. In terms of how to carry out informal assessments with these patients, we recommend applying a structured approach to testing hypotheses, based on what you see at each stage of the interaction. This is more around 'how' to approach assessment rather than a strict task-list of 'what' to do as the start-point and stages will vary according to factors such as location, environment, the patient's presentation (e.g. are their eyes open or closed? Are they seated in a chair or lying in bed? Are there behavioural signs of agitation or is their presentation calm and still?). Nevertheless, given psychologists' training in structured behavioural assessment and the scientist–practitioner approach, this creative approach to testing what the patient can and can't do via a bespoke hypothesis testing approach may be a better use of our skills than using formal assessment tools, particularly when other members of the team are confident in administering the CRS-R, WHIM, and/or SMART.

The following list contains examples of things to think about during the assessment process. It is not intended to be exhaustive, but rather to encourage a curious and creative approach to assessment. It is also not discipline-specific. As referred to earlier, a team approach is vital, and allocating different questions to different team members and/or doing joint sessions is likely to be of far higher value than each member of the team carrying out a unidisciplinary assessment in isolation. It is likely that close teamworking between SLT, OT, and neuropsychology will be of particular value, although joint working with physiotherapy, nurses, medics/rehabilitation doctors and, where available, music therapists may also occur. Some additional guidance and means of capturing informal team assessment findings can be found in the Putney PDOC Toolkit (Wilford et al, 2019), which can be downloaded from the website of the Royal Hospital for Neuro-disability (www.rhn.org.uk).

Questions to consider:

- Is there any difference in response to photographs of family/friends versus famous people who were of interest to the patient, versus strangers?
- What about between audio or video recordings of the same groups of people?
- What about reactions to pets or other animals?
- When you go outside, do they react to changes in the weather, the feeling of the sun on their face, the sounds, sights, and smells of nature?
- Do they show reactions to emotionally salient stimuli e.g. different facial expressions, the sounds of laughing and crying, or slapstick comedy?
- Do they show reactions to music e.g. previously favourite songs/pieces of music compared with genres or pieces they didn't like?
- In collaboration with SLT colleagues (who can advise on safety), are there reactions to different tastes, including past likes and dislikes?
- For patients who do not have a tracheostomy, are there reactions to different smells, including past likes and dislikes (if known) and familiar versus unfamiliar smells?

- What reactions (if any) do they show to touch from different types of stimuli, e.g. hard versus soft, light versus heavy, warm versus cold, familiar items versus unfamiliar?
- Do they show more behaviours or higher-level behaviours if you vary the setting, who is present and/or their physical position (lying, sitting, standing)?

8.2.3 Assessing for evidence of emergence from PDOC

Whilst some people will remain in a PDOC for the rest of their lives, the operational criteria for determining that a person has 'emerged' from PDOC, i.e. that they no longer present with disordered consciousness, are described earlier in this chapter, along with some of the criticisms of current criteria. Detailed descriptions of how to establish emergence can be found in annex 1a of the RCP guidelines, which is available as a free download. These include examples of objects, questions, and objects that might be used to assess functional object use, yes/no reliability, and discriminatory choice-making from a choice of two. However, rather than focus rigidly on whether a patient has 'passed' any of these thresholds, we recommend a broader approach to structured assessment of cognition as outlined in Chapter 4, looking to determine any islets of ability against a background of severe global impairment.

8.3 Diagnosis, formulation, and monitoring

The team aim is to arrive at both an accurate diagnosis of the person's condition and a thorough formulation of what they can and cannot do across a range of settings. As described in Chapter 9, people with LIS are essential to differentiate from people with PDOC. The diagnosis is effectively a label of whether the person is in VS, MCS−, MCS+ or whether they have emerged from PDOC and although this is important, it is not sufficient to determine prognosis, nor to guide management and intervention strategies. The team's more thorough formulation is a much broader description encompassing the range of behaviours the person has shown and the specific stimuli and environments which are most likely to elicit responses; this informs programmes for ongoing management which are outlined in more detail below. We have found that neuropsychologists' input can be valuable in helping knit the broader formulation together, and in challenging the group think and team narrative when needed. For example, in PDOC as in other conditions, it is common for assumptions to be made and, on occasion, for these to go unchallenged and/or for the most confident voice in the team to dominate. Facilitating a team culture and atmosphere in which challenge is viewed positively is vital, alongside a willingness to work together to test things out.

Monitoring of the person's awareness and responsiveness over time using both formal and informal assessments is essential. This is partly because of the importance of the trajectory of change in determining prognosis, but also because identifying any changes in rehabilitation potential is crucial in ensuring timely access to specialist therapy, both to facilitate any changes in functioning and to enhance quality of life. Discussions around the most appropriate ways to monitor for change or lack of it are an essential part of teamwork.

8.4 The role of EEG and functional imaging

An in-depth discussion of electrophysiological and functional imaging techniques is beyond the scope of the current chapter but it is important for clinicians to be aware that this is a rapidly changing field in which the evidence-base is growing. One of the groundbreaking studies in this area was the use of fMRI to detect awareness in people previously presumed to be in VS by imagining either playing tennis or moving around in their home (Owen et al. 2006). There is undoubted evidence that a small percentage of patients who present behaviourally as being in PDOC can nevertheless show signs of awareness via EEG or functional imaging, including the ability to follow commands (e.g. Cruse et al., 2011), or even communicate basic yes/no responses (e.g. Monti et al., 2010). Although most patients who are able to generate such responses do develop the ability to show responses behaviourally over time (see Pan et al., 2020), it is possible that wider adaptation of such techniques in the future might enable these patients to be identified earlier in the pathway. How these findings can be used in rehabilitation settings is not established. Not everyone will be able to go into a scanner because of metalwork associated with treatment for trauma and we cannot put people in a scanner to ask questions such as what clothes they wish to wear that day. Furthermore, it is not clear in the context of so much brain damage what can be extrapolated from this very basic level of response. Families are noted to attribute a 'special significance of "brain scans"' as providing some unique and conclusive information compared to the standard behavioural-based diagnostic assessment (Cruse et al., 2024). As discussed further in Chapter 4, there is a risk that evidence of 'some' intact cognition is interpreted as meaning that all cognition is intact, when this is highly unlikely to be the case.

At present, within a clinical setting in the UK, the most likely opportunity for patients in PDOC to access such EEG or functional imaging techniques (such as fMRI) would be via a research paradigm with appropriate ethical approval. Such ethical approval typically involves consultation with patients' families given that these patients cannot provide informed consent, and clinicians should therefore be prepared for the scenario of such protocols being available, and of supporting families' expectations.

8.5 Emotion-related behaviours

As described earlier in this chapter, patients in PDOC, even those in VS, can show emotion-related behaviours such as laughing, tears and grimacing.

We have used the phrase 'emotion-related behaviours' deliberately in order to highlight that careful assessment is needed to determine whether such behaviours are indeed likely to be regulated by the patient's internal emotional state, or whether they are occurring spontaneously with no evidence of being contingent on thoughts and feelings. We have encountered many instances of care teams and families assuming that behaviours such as tears, grimaces, and incoherent vocalisations must be indicative of depression and require urgent intervention. As outlined in more detail in Chapter 6 on assessment of mood in severe brain injury, a personalised approach to assessment, formulation and monitoring is needed in this patient group. This involves looking at the frequency and intensity of the target behaviour, the circumstances in which it arises, and any other emotion-related behaviours that may not have been flagged; for example, the formulation for a patient who shows frequent episodes of tears, sobbing and grimacing in the absence of any episodes of smiling and laughing will be different from that of a patient who shows infrequent episodes of tears in the context of frequent observations of smiling. This behaviour-based approach is needed since, by definition, patients in PDOC lack a reliable and consistent form of communication, and therefore any responses to even a simple self-report tool (e.g. those which involve pointing at a stimulus or answering yes/no questions) will not be valid, and observer-rating scales should also be approached with extreme caution (Rose et al., 2022).

Without a patient-centred assessment process, there are risks that medications such as anti-depressants may be prescribed to these patients in the absence of a clear baseline, formulation, and monitoring plan. It is important to note that in the absence of reliable self-report data, monitoring must not only encompass the behaviours that are being targeted for change (e.g. to reduce tearfulness) but also any potential undesirable effects (e.g. a reduction in wakefulness or cognitively mediated behaviours, or development of physical side-effects).

8.6 Behaviours that challenge

Patients in PDOC may have active movements, which can result in behaviours that can cause risk to self or others. These risks may include trachestomy or feeding (PEG/JEG/NG) tubes being dislodged, bedding covers being kicked off, smearing of faeces, repetitive scratching of the skin, and limbs moving with staff potentially being hit or kicked during care tasks. The risks of assuming that such behaviours are cognitively mediated, and the steps needed to undertake a thorough objective assessment are described in more detail in Chapter 5. However, it is important to highlight that these risks are particularly high in this most severely impaired patient group, and that very careful consideration of the least restrictive ways to manage behaviours in best interests is needed, particularly if measures such as physical restraints (like mittens or abdominal binders) are judged necessary.

At the most severe end of PDOC, a patient in a vegetative state may show an almost total absence of spontaneous behaviour other than eye-opening (although of course reflexive behaviours like moving, sneezing, startling to loud noises, and crying can all be present). For these patients, observers may develop beliefs analogous with a 'sleeping beauty' idea, in which the gross absence of behaviour is assumed to mean that there is nothing wrong with the brain, and that the patient just needs to 'wake up' and then everything will be fine. This is highly unlikely to be the case, although this assumption has also been fostered by movies and media coverage (Wijdicks & Wijdicks, 2006) of PDOC, sometimes with explicit reference to sleeping beauty (Samuel & Kitzinger, 2013). This erroneous belief can lead to attempts by people who care for the patient to attempt to find the right key, piece of music, visitor or item that enables the patient to 'wake'. We have seen families say hurtful things and do hurtful things to the patient as they are so wedded to the idea that they can 'shock' the person awake. There can also be challenges to the diagnosis if observers assume that patients in VS may have locked-in-syndrome – i.e. an assumption that the absence of behaviour is due to disruption to the motor pathways in the context of intact cognition (see Chapter 9 on LIS). These assumptions can persist in part because the lack of behaviour also means that there is no definitive observable proof of absence of intent; addressing these assumptions then forms part of the systematic team based assessment of PDOC as described earlier in this chapter.

Although some of these patients may show no change in behavioural repertoire, others may demonstrate a wider range of behaviour over time due primarily to some spontaneous recovery. When patients in PDOC start to emerge, in our experience it is often the case that any behaviour is interpreted as a positive indicator of change, both in terms of interpretation of the behaviour (e.g. 'he wanted a drink' rather than 'he has developed spontaneous but non-purposeful movement in his arms'), and potentially in terms of biased reporting of either 'good' or 'bad' behaviours whilst ignoring or downplaying other behaviours. The full profile of behaviour can get missed if there is too much focus on one area, which leads in turn to less than optimal care. For example, prescribing medication to reduce the frequency of a 'bad' behaviour may also reduce the frequency of 'good' and desirable behaviours. Thus, a thorough assessment and formulation is vital, and joint sessions/hypothesis testing and psychoeducation may be beneficial with both teams and families to promote a collaborative understanding.

8.7 Intervention and management strategies

Once the diagnosis and formulation are clear, there is a need for an ongoing management/intervention programme that will optimise the person's arousal (sleep/wake cycle), physical condition and quality of life and provide opportunities for any further changes in awareness behaviour and responsiveness to be identified promptly. The focus of the team is on working to manage the range of disabilities the person has such as seating, bed positioning, spasticity, splinting, optimising health conditions, and controlling the environment etc. The idea is that this will enable the person to be most well and enable the brain to make any spontaneous recovery it can.

A key principle in designing a management plan is sensory regulation. There is sometimes a desire to bombard these patients with constant stimuli in the hope that something will elicit a response and almost 'pull' the patient out of PDOC. Whilst this desire is understandable, a regulation approach, interspersing active tasks with periods of much lower sensory stimulation, is generally recommended. It is for these reasons that clinical areas will have times during the day of low sound, low lighting, and low activity so that the brain rests and is not overwhelmed. The clinical reasoning of sensory stimulation programmes is to create conditions to optimize cortical activity and therefore neuroplasticity through the environment and stimulation. Too little stimulation is problematic as it may limit plasticity, too much stimulation is equally problematic as the person may habituate to it. Therefore, it is important that a sensory stimulation programme exposes a person to differentiated stimuli and in a controlled and balanced way. Although the evidence-base is limited, prioritizing stimuli with emotional salience and/or autobiographical relevance is supported (Abbate et al., 2014), and a multi-modal approach is also recommended (Padilla & Domina, 2016). Stimuli must be chosen to fit with the person's ability to process sensory information – e.g. visual stimuli should be avoided if the patient is blind, olfactory stimuli should be avoided if the patient breathes through a tracheostomy tube. A creative approach should also be taken such that stimuli are varied. For example, if a patient responds to auditory stimuli, then a programme may encompass favourite music, recordings of their family talking about special memories and events, and things of personal relevance where appropriate such as religious readings (e.g. from the Bible, Quran) but thought should also be given to include sounds the person would have heard in their daily life (e.g. kettles, microwaves, animal, and traffic sounds). The same principles apply to other senses (tactile, gustatory, olfactory, visual). Involving family in generating ideas and contributing items can be valuable both in terms of personalising the programme for the person, and in giving family members, particularly children, a sense of active involvement in the patient's day-to-day life, including ideas for activities they can do themselves when visiting. It is important also to note that episodes of active care such as hoisting or showering are examples of high sensory overload tasks and therefore a period of reduced stimulation should be scheduled immediately after each one.

Such programmes build on the observations made during the informal, personalised assessments of any behaviours shown by the person, particularly any emotion-related behaviours that are typically associated with pleasure and also any activities that are particularly helpful to families. For example, if family members find it helpful to read to the patient, or tell their brain-injured parent what they have done at school, or rub hand-cream into the patient's skin, then these types of activities should be built into the programme whether or not the patient shows signs of recognition or pleasure, provided that there are no signs of distress.

8.8 Working with families

Families and friends of people in PDOC have experienced a devastating change in their lives too, and it is not expected that any of them will find it easy to adjust to the person's brain injury and the impact of this on every aspect of life. The importance of involving families in discussions and joint sessions has been threaded through the sections of this chapter, and this close involvement is always important for those families who wish to be engage with it. However, some families choose not to do so, whether this is because the pressures and distractions of daily life are too great in a context in which they know the person with the brain injury is being well cared for, or whether they simply cannot face the emotional stress at this period of time. Some families will view the PDOC as a loss of the 'person' before they actually die. This is highlighted by the gravestone of Terri Schiavo in the USA, whose life and PDOC had a great deal of media coverage. Her gravestone encapsulates the challenge for those who love the person and provides three dates: 'born' (her birth date), 'departed' (the date of her brain injury) and 'at peace' (the date of actual her physical death). This sense of the person having gone after their brain injury, but yet also still physically being present, is a unique form of loss which has been termed Ambiguous Loss (Boss, 2000) and is discussed in Chapter 10. As PDOC is so rare, most family members will be learning about it, and it can be helpful to signpost families to the Coma and Disorders of Consciousness (CDOC) Research Centre and Healthtalk.org, which have resources on diagnosis, treatment decisions, legal processes, and includes video clips of families describing their experiences. Kitzinger & Kitzinger (2014) highlight respecting the range of ways families will cope with such an unusual situation. Specific guidance on how to provide psychological support to families is discussed in Chapter 10.

8.9 Mental capacity and best interests

General principles around mental capacity and best interests were outlined earlier in Chapter 2. Whilst both the MCA (2005) and the Code of Practice (2007) state that capacity is decision-specific and not based on diagnosis, it is nevertheless the case that when a person has a PDOC diagnosis, they will lack capacity for all decisions in their lives (consent to care and treatment, where they live, managing their property and financial affairs etc). This is because a diagnosis of PDOC by definition is characterised by an absence of any form of reliable and consistent communication, and it is consequently impossible for them to demonstrate understanding, retention and weighing up of information. Even the very limited choice making that can be seen in patients with MCS+ cannot be assumed to be capacitous; for example, if a patient selects a banana-flavoured yoghurt from a choice of banana versus strawberry in an SLT session then it does not necessarily follow that the patient understood the options on offer and made a specific selection based on preference – they may simply have chosen the item on the left, or the one with the most eye-catching container. This is a concrete in the moment and visually, olfactory and verbally supported choice. It is fundamentally different to an abstract, future focussed conversation containing multiple factors to weigh up.

For this group of patients, unless their awareness and ability to communicate responses improves, the focus of applying the MCA is less about maximising supported decision-making and analysing unwise versus incapacitious decisions, and more about best interests decision-making. Best interests decision-making applies to all areas of care, which means that the person's daily care plan should be constructed with family involvement to encompass factors such as whether the person preferred a shower versus a flannel wash, what clothes they liked to wear, how they prefer their hair to be washed and styled, and whether they preferred to have facial hair or be clean-shaven and so on.

Best interests decision-making also applies to all aspects of treatment escalation planning and administering of life-sustaining treatments, including clinically assisted nutrition and hydration (CANH). This is an emotionally and ethically demanding area of practice (Olgiati et al., 2023). Detailed descriptions of the process of best interests decision-making around ongoing CANH were outlined in Chapter 2, as this applies to ALL patients who lack capacity (also see The British Psychological Society 2021, Supporting people who lack mental capacity – a guide to best interests decision making). Nevertheless, this is a particularly pertinent issue for patients in PDOC, and most of the cases that have been heard in the courts have involved people with a PDOC diagnosis. Kitzinger and Kitzinger (2013) described that there is rarely an overt choice between death or recovery, and the reality is a continuum of things in-between. Families grapple with what the person would have wanted in their situation and as the prognosis becomes more obvious over time, the opportunities to stop life sustaining treatment decline as the person becomes more medically stable.

Some clinicians will wish to delay difficult conversations because of concerns about the family's readiness to consider this, or indeed their own discomfort with addressing profoundly difficult conversations about life and living and death and dying. The very nature of introducing this topic for families who are beginning to adjust to a new reality brings a level of uncertainty, not only about whether their loved one may yet die, but also about their relationships with the staff looking after their loved one. Our advice is to open a conversation about this early to provide a foundation for understanding that even if the best interest decision is to continue CANH, regular treatment reviews are legally required. This helps families grapple with the concept that prognosis is about probabilities, not certainties and different decisions could be made in the future.

For many families, there is also a distinction between the idea of removing treatment which will have an inevitable outcome of death, and the process of this death. Death that occurs following removal of nutrition and hydration is not an event, but a process, and it takes time. Families are often very distressed by this process and perceive it as unnecessarily long and protracted. From a legal perspective, there is a difference between the removal of a futile treatment (that is not aiding recovery) and a deliberate act to end a person's life (euthanasia), but families often report that this legal distinction is irrelevant emotionally. This may feel even more distressing when the best interest decision is disputed by the family and imposed by a Court of Protection judgement. For some families, a judgement may be more helpful as it places the responsibility on a neutral expert (the judge) rather than on the family and the clinical team that they have got to know and formed views about. Irrespective of any best interest decision, all outcomes are distressing because all solutions are 'bad' when the context is that something devastating has happened. This means supporting families throughout the process is vital, as discussed in more detail in Chapter 10.

References

Abbate, C., Trimarchi, P. D., Basile, I., Mazzucchi, A., & Devalle, G. (2014). Sensory stimulation for patients with disorders of consciousness: From stimulation to rehabilitation. *Frontiers in Human Neuroscience, 8*, 616. https://doi.org/10.3389/fnhum.2014.00616

Bruno, M. A., Fernández-Espejo, D., Lehembre, R., Tshibanda, L., Vanhaudenhuyse, A., Gosseries, O., Lommers, E., Napolitani, M., Noirhomme, Q., Boly, M., Papa, M., Owen, A., Maquet, P., Laureys, S., & Soddu, A. (2011). Multimodal neuroimaging in patients with disorders of consciousness showing "functional hemispherectomy". *Progress in Brain Research, 193*, 323–333. https://doi.org/10.1016/B978-0-444-53839-0.00021-1

Cruse, D., Chennu, S., Chatelle, C., Bekinschtein, T. A., Fernández-Espejo, D., Pickard, J. D., Laureys, S., & Owen, A. M. (2011). Bedside detection of awareness in the vegetative state: A cohort study. *Lancet (London, England), 378*(9809), 2088–2094. https://doi.org/10.1016/S0140-6736(11)61224-5

Cruse, D., Ragazinskaite, K., Chinner, A., Bareham, C., Roberts, N., Banner, R., Chennu, S., & Villa, D. (2024). Family caregivers' sense-making of the results of functional neurodiagnostics for patients with Prolonged Disorders of Consciousness. *Neuropsychological Rehabilitation, 34*(9), 1257–1278. https://doi.org/10.1080/09602011.2023.2299448

da Conceição Teixeira, L., Blacker, D., Campos, C., Garrett, C., Duport, S., & Rocha, N. B. (2021). Repeated clinical assessment using sensory modality assessment and rehabilitation technique for diagnosis in prolonged disorders of consciousness. *Frontiers in Human Neuroscience, 15*, 728637. https://doi.org/10.3389/fnhum.2021.728637

Department of Health. (2005). Mental Capacity Act. London: HMSO.

Dhamapurkar, S. K., Rose, A., Florschutz, G., & Wilson, B. A. (2016). The natural history of continuing improvement in an individual after a long period of impaired consciousness: The story of I.J. *Brain Injury, 30*(2), 230–236. https://doi.org/10.3109/02699052.2015.1094132

Elliott, L., Coleman, M., Shiel, A., Wilson, B.A., Badwan, D., Menon, D., & Pickard, J. (2005). Effect of posture on levels of arousal and awareness in vegetative and minimally conscious states: A preliminary investigation. *Journal of Neurology, Neurosurgery and Psychiatry, 76*, 298–299.

Giacino, J. T., Ashwal, S., Childs, N., Cranford, R., Jennett, B., Katz, D. I., Kelly, J. P., Rosenberg, J. H., Whyte, J., Zafonte, R. D., & Zasler, N. D. (2002). The minimally conscious state: Definition and diagnostic criteria. *Neurology, 58*(3), 349–353. https://doi.org/10.1212/wnl.58.3.349

Giacino, J. T., Kalmar, K., & Whyte, J. (2004). The JFK Coma Recovery Scale-Revised: Measurement characteristics and diagnostic utility. *Archives of physical medicine and rehabilitation, 85*(12), 2020–2029. https://doi.org/10.1016/j.apmr.2004.02.033

Giacino, J. T., Katz, D. I., Schiff, N. D., Whyte, J., Ashman, E. J., Ashwal, S., Barbano, R., Hammond, F. M., Laureys, S., Ling, G. S. F., Nakase-Richardson, R., Seel, R. T., Yablon, S., Getchius, T. S. D., Gronseth, G. S., & Armstrong, M. J. (2018). Practice guideline update recommendations summary: Disorders of consciousness: Report of the Guideline Development, Dissemination, and Implementation Subcommittee of the American Academy of Neurology; the American Congress of Rehabilitation Medicine; and the National Institute on Disability, Independent Living, and Rehabilitation Research. *Neurology, 91*(10), 450–460. https://doi.org/10.1212/WNL.0000000000005926

Gill-Thwaites, H., & Munday, R. (2004). The Sensory Modality Assessment and Rehabilitation Technique (SMART): A valid and reliable assessment for vegetative state and minimally conscious state patients. *Brain Injury*, 18(12):1255–69.

Hammond, F. M., Giacino, J., Nakase Richardon R., Sherer, M., Zafonte, R. D., Whytem J., et al (2019). Disorders of consciousness due to traumatic brain injury: Functional status ten years post-injury. *Journal of Neurotrauma, 36* (7), 1136–1146. https://doi.org/10.1089/neu.2018.5954

Illman, N. A., & Crawford, S. (2018). Late-recovery from 'permanent' vegetative state in the context of severe traumatic brain injury: A case report exploring objective and subjective aspects of recovery and rehabilitation. *Neuropsychological Rehabilitation, 28*(8), 1360–1374. https://doi.org/10.1080/09602011.2017.1313167

Kitzinger, C., & Kitzinger J. (2014). Grief, anger and despair in relatives of severely brain injured patients: Responding without pathologising. *Clinical Rehabilitation, 28*(7), 627–631. doi:10.1177/0269215514527844

Kitzinger, J. & Kitzinger, C. (2013). The 'window of opportunity' for death after severe brain injury: Family experiences. *Sociology of Health and Illness, 35*(7), 1095–1112. doi:10.1111/1467-9566.12020

Laureys, S., Celesia, G. G., Cohadon, F., Lavrijsen, J., León-Carrión, J., Sannita, W. G., Sazbon, L., Schmutzhard, E., von Wild, K. R., Zeman, A., Dolce, G., & European Task Force on Disorders of Consciousness (2010). Unresponsive wakefulness syndrome: A new name for the vegetative state or apallic syndrome. *BMC Medicine, 8*, 68. https://doi.org/10.1186/1741-7015-8-68

Magee, W. L., Siegert, R. J., Daveson, B. A., Lenton-Smith, G., & Taylor, S. M. (2014). Music therapy assessment tool for awareness in disorders of consciousness (MATADOC): Standardisation of the principal subscale to assess awareness in patients with disorders of consciousness. *Neuropsychological Rehabilitation, 24*(1), 101–124.

Monti, M. M, Vanhaudenhuyse, A., Coleman, M. R., Boly, M., Pickard, J. D., Tshibanda, L., Owen, A. M., & Laureys, S. (2010). Willful modulation of brain activity in disorders of consciousness. *The New England Journal of Medicine, 18*;362(7):579–89. doi:10.1056/NEJMoa0905370

Nakamura, Y., Shiozaki, T., Ito, H., Nakao S., Ogura, H & Oda, J. (2023). Long-term outcomes over 20 years in persons with persistent disorders of consciousness after traumatic brain injury. *Neurotrauma Reports, 4*(1), 805–812. doi:10.1089/neur.2023.0080

Nakase-Richardson, R., Yablon, S. A., Sherer, M., Evans, C. C., & Nick, T. G. (2008). Serial yes/no reliability after traumatic brain injury: implications regarding the operational criteria for emergence from the minimally conscious state. *Journal of Neurology, Neurosurgery, and Psychiatry, 79*(2), 216–218. https://doi.org/10.1136/jnnp.2007.127795

Office of the Public Guardian. (2007). Mental Capacity Act Code of Practice. https://assets.publishing.service.gov.uk/media/5f6cc6138fa8f541f6763295/Mental-capacity-act-code-of-practice.pdf

Olgiati, E., Hinchliffe, J., Hanrahan, A., Mantovani, P. & Crawford, S. (2023). Ethical and practical issues for the psychologist working with patients in a disorder of consciousness (p. 331–347). In: In Fish, J., Betteridge, S., & Wilson, B.A. (Eds.). (2023). Rare Conditions, Diagnostic Challenges, and Controversies in Clinical Neuropsychology: Out of the Ordinary (1st ed.). Routledge.

Owen, A. M., Coleman, M. R., Boly, M., Davis, M. H., Laureys, S., & Pickard, J. D. (2006). Detecting awareness in the vegetative state. *Science, 313*(5792), 1402. https://doi.org/10.1126/science.1130197

Padilla, R. & Domina, A., (2016). Effectiveness of sensory stimulation to improve arousal and alertness of people in a coma or persistent vegetative state after traumatic brain injury: A systematic review. *American Journal of Occupational Therapy, 70*(3), 1–8. doi:10.5014/ajot.2016.021022

Pan, J., Xie, Q., Qin, P., Chen, Y., He, Y., Huang, H., Wang, F., Ni, X., Cichocki, A., Yu, R., Li, Y. (2020). Prognosis for patients with cognitive motor dissociation identified by brain-computer interface. *Brain, 143*(4):1177–1189. doi:10.1093/brain/awaa026

Pundole, A., & Crawford, S. (2018). The assessment of language and the emergence from disorders of consciousness. *Neuropsychological Rehabilitation, 28*(8), 1285–1294. doi:10.1080/09602011.2017.1307766

Pundole, A., Varley, R., & Beeke, S. (2021). Assessing emergence from a prolonged disorder of consciousness: Current opinion and practice in the UK. *Neuropsychological Rehabilitation, 31* (7), 1003–1027. https://doi.org/10.1080/09602011.2020.1758160

Rose, A.E., Cullen, B., Crawford, S., & Evans, J. J. (2022). A systematic review of mood and depression measures in people with severe cognitive and communication impairments following acquired brain injury. *Clinical Rehabilitation, 37*(5):679–700. doi:10.1177/02692155221139023

Royal College of Physicians. (2020). *Prolonged disorders of consciousness following sudden onset brain injury: National clinical guidelines*. RCP.

Samuel, G., & Kitzinger, J. (2013). Reporting consciousness in coma: Media framing of neuro-scientific research, hope, and the response of families with relatives in vegetative and minimally conscious states. *JOMEC Journal*, *3*, 10244. doi:10.18573/j.2013.10244

Schnakers, C., Vanhaudenhuyse, A., Giacino, J., Ventura, M., Boly, M., Majerus, S., Moonen, G., & Laureys S. (2009). Diagnostic accuracy of the vegetative and minimally conscious state: Clinical consensus versus standardized neurobehavioral assessment. *BMC Neurology 9*. doi:10.1186/1471-2377-9-35

Scolding, N., Owen, A. M., & Keown, J. (2021). Prolonged disorders of consciousness: a critical evaluation of the new UK guidelines. *Brain: a Journal of Neurology*, *144*(6), 1655–1660. https://doi.org/10.1093/brain/awab063

Shiel, A., Horn, S.A., Wilson, B.A., Watson, M.J., Campbell, M.J. & McLellan, D. L., (2000). The Wessex Head Injury Matrix (WHIM) main scale: a preliminary report on a scale to assess and monitor patient recovery after severe head injury. *Clinical Rehabilitation*, *14*(4), 408–416. doi:10.1191/0269215500cr326oa

Stokes, V., Gunn, S., Schouwenaars, K., & Badwan, D. (2018). Neurobehavioural assessment and diagnosis in disorders of consciousness: a preliminary study of the Sensory Tool to Assess Responsiveness (STAR). *Neuropsychological Rehabilitation*, *28*(6), 966–983. https://doi.org/10.1080/09602011.2016.1214604

Turner-Stokes, L., Bassett, P., Rose, H., Ashford, S., & Thu, A. (2015). Serial measurement of Wessex Head Injury Matrix in the diagnosis of patients in vegetative and minimally conscious states: A cohort analysis. *BMJ Open*, *5*(4), e006051. https://doi.org/10.1136/bmjopen-2014-006051

Wade, D. (2018). How many patients in a prolonged disorder of consciousness might need a best interests meeting about starting or continuing gastrostomy feeding? *Clinical Rehabilitation*, *32* (11), 1551–1564. https://doi.org/10.1177/0269215518777285

Wang, J., Hu, X., Hu, Z., Sun, Z., Laureys, S., & Di, H. (2020). The misdiagnosis of prolonged disorders of consciousness by a clinical consensus compared with repeated coma-recovery scale-revised assessment. *BMC Neurology*, *20*(1), 343. https://doi.org/10.1186/s12883-020-01924-9

Wijdicks, E. F., & Wijdicks, C. A. (2006). The portrayal of coma in contemporary motion pictures. *Neurology*, *66*(9), 1300–1303. doi:10.1212/01.wnl.0000210497.62202.e9

Wilford, S., Pundole, A., Crawford, S., & Hanrahan A. (2019). The putney prolonged disorders of consciousness toolkit. www.rhn.org.uk/wp-content/uploads/2019/05/Putney-PDoC-toolkit-v1.0-WEB.pdf

Wilson, B. A., Dhamapurkar, S., Tunnard, C., Watson, P., & Florschutz, G. (2013). The effect of positioning on the level of arousal and awareness in patients in the vegetative state or the minimally conscious state: A replication and extension of a previous finding. *Brain Impairment*, *14*(3), 475–479. https://doi.org/10.1017/BrImp.2013.34

Yelden, K., Duport, S., James, L. M., Kempny, A., Farmer, S. F., Leff, A. P., & Playford, E. D. (2018). Late recovery of awareness in prolonged disorders of consciousness – A cross-sectional cohort study. *Disability Rehabilitation*, *40*(20), 2433–2438. https://doi.org/10.1080/09638288.2017.1339209

9   Working with people with locked in syndrome

Locked in syndrome (LIS) is a neurological condition caused by damage to the brainstem (to the ventral pons and caudal midbrain) following trauma, haemorrhage, or an ischemic occlusion to the basiliar artery (Halan et al., 2021) or masses, infections, or demyelination (Das et al., 2023), but without causing damage to other areas of the brain which are associated with cognition (Smith & Delargey, 2005). The person is conscious, aware, able to see, hear, and think, but is left unable to speak or move, with paralysis of nearly all their voluntary muscles, and hence is 'locked' inside their body and unable to alert others to their situation (Laureys et al., 2005). People typically retain the ability to move their eyes vertically but not horizontally and, at times, are still able to deliberately blink (Schnakers et al., 2008). The very limited range of purposeful movements the person can deliberately make means that recognising the condition is challenging; misdiagnosis can occur, including assuming the person is unaware of themselves and the world around them and unable to think, such as in a prolonged disorder of consciousness (PDOC). Indeed, the challenges around diagnosis mean that it is common for families rather than clinicians to be the first to realise that the person is aware, with 2.5 months on average needed to establish a diagnosis of LIS, and distressing reports of patients being in this state for several years before their awareness was recognised (Laureys et al., 2005).

Early descriptions consistent with the modern diagnosis of LIS were published in novels such as Dumas' 'The Count of Monte Cristo' in the nineteenth century, although the first clinical descriptions and the coining of the term 'locked-in-syndrome' are associated with Plum and Posner in the early 1970's. Subsequently, three main types of LIS were identified based on specific physical presentations in the context of presumed intact cognition (Bauer et al., 1979). In Classic LIS, a person has intact consciousness, a complete loss of the motor ability to create speech (anarthria), complete inability to move their body (tetraplegia), and voluntary movement control only over their vertical eye movements. In people with Incomplete or Partial LIS, some additional limited voluntary movement is also possible, such as finger movement or mouth movement. In contrast, people with Total LIS have no movement control at all, including of the eyes. To date, the only way to identify any cortical functions in Total LIS is through functional imaging

DOI: 10.4324/9781032665986-9

or EEG techniques (Schnakers et al., 2009). In both Classic and Incomplete LIS forms, blink response or eye movement–response to questions can be used to identify consciousness (Das et al., 2023).

Once someone is diagnosed with LIS, it is typically a life-long condition. A recent review by Halan et al. (2021) noted that the associated medical complexities resulted in most people with LIS dying within the first year (87% in the first 4 months). As would be expected from the diagnostic criteria, patients with LIS present with profound disabilities. The absence of voluntary limb movements does not just impact their mobility but also renders them dependent on others for all care, including such simple tasks as turning in bed, scratching an itch, or adjusting the position of their feet on the footplate of their wheelchair. Patients are typically doubly incontinent, may require a tracheostomy or even a ventilator to support breathing, and are dependent on a feeding tube for nutrition and hydration. Some changes in the class of LIS can occur with neurorehabilitation, typically early post-injury, but not usually to a level of functional independence (Hocker & Wijdicks 2015). In a series of 14 patients, some motor recovery was reported within 6 months of injury in 21% of the sample, i.e. 3 of the 14 patients (Casanova et al., 2003). The same study found that ventilation was weaned in half of the sample, swallowing returned in 42%, bladder and bowel control returned in 35%, and communication gains were seen in terms of both verbal communication gains (28%) or communication through devices (42%). For those who do survive the first year, there was a 5-year survival rate of 86%, with a 10-year survival rate of 80% (Halan et al., 2021), indicating that for those who survive the first year following injury, there is a chronicity to living with LIS.

LIS is rare. The average age of occurrence is between the ages of 30 and 50 (Das et al., 2023), but it has also been recorded in children (Bruno et al., 2009). It is not straightforward to establish international prevalence of LIS. Using published information on people living with LIS and national population data, estimates of prevalence were made as displayed.

Country	France	Norway	USA
Number of people per million with LIS	7 people per million	9 people per million	3 people per million
Derivation of information	500 people in LIS society, in a population of 67.75 million (2021)	51 people on a National register, in a population of 5.43 million (2021)	1000 people in a population of 331.9 million (2021)

(Continued)

Country	France	Norway	USA
Reference	Schnetzer et al. (2023)	Nilsen et al. (2023)	[https://rared iseases.info. nih.gov/disea ses/6919/ locked-in-syndrome Feb 2024]

When a patient presents with tetraplegia and anarthria, early optimisation of their physical status is key. This includes optimising medical stability and pharmacological interventions, postural and skin management both in a suitable specialist wheelchair and in bed, and management of incontinence, any interventions to support breathing, and nutritional status. Whilst sensation, including pain, may be absent or diminished (Das et al., 2023), it should nevertheless be investigated as part of the medical examination. In scenarios where these physical issues have been challenging to manage in the acute service or other referral setting, they will be priorities for the professional team in the neurorehabilitation setting. The other major priority, which is likely to be focussed on in parallel to physical management rather than subsequent to it, is to establish a means of communication. In LIS, speech is not possible due to anarthria caused by paralysis of the facial-glosso-pharyngo-laryngeal muscles and damage of the corticobulbar fibres (Yokose et al., 2018). Therefore, reliance on the only aspect of deliberate and voluntary control the person retains, of their eyes, is needed. Typically, the ability to look up (vertical gaze) is preserved in the rostral portion of the midbrain (Patterson & Grabois, 1986). However, vision itself can be affected with reports of double vision (diplopia), blurred vision, and medial and lateral gaze palsies (Wilson et al., 2011; Yokose et al., 2018). Other conditions affecting the eyes such as ptosis or nystagmus can also affect communication and require careful investigation. More prosaically, checking whether the patient is long- or short-sighted and needs glasses must not be missed out. Overall, it is important to establish the person's visual and hearing abilities, and any interventions or aids needed to support these, as early as possible in the assessment process.

As described above, there is a risk that patients with LIS may be misdiagnosed as being in a disorder of consciousness. However, the opposite problem has also been reported, in which patients who present with tetraplegia and anarthria in the context of severely or profoundly impaired cognition have been described as being in LIS in spite of their extensive cognitive impairments (Crawford et al., 2023). The term 'locked in plus syndrome' ('LiPS') has been suggested to describe the subset of these patients who present with such profound impairments that they are in a disorder of consciousness, in whom the neurological damage extends beyond the pons and into the thalamus (Schnetzer et al., 2023).

Given the risks associated with diagnostic errors of either kind, it is vital for all patients presenting with profound physical impairments to have their communicative abilities thoroughly assessed. This assessment process will usually be led by a specialist speech and language therapist (SLT). However, the complexity of this patient group means that additional input from one or more other disciplines with relevant skills in understanding cognition, positioning, and assistive technology may be helpful. The aim is to determine whether the patient can demonstrate at least one form of reliable communication strategy.

Investigation of a person's communicative ability must explore whether they are able to reliably and consistently respond to questions across time. The techniques used to do this are described in more detail in Chapter 4; however, they must initially involve closed questions, which can be answered by eye pointing (to stimuli held one above another due to the vertical only eye movement) or to yes/no questions. The principles of counterbalancing and checking for above chance responding using binomial statistics are necessary before more comprehensive communication methods are introduced.

Once patients have shown that they have awareness and some ability to communicate, SLTs and other members of the team will work to determine whether the patient can learn to use any other methods, with eye gaze, Alphabet charts, E-tran eye gaze systems among the augmentative-assisted communication devices (Lugo et al., 2015) commonly used. Using eye movements and an alphabet chart, the person with LIS is shown or hears letters and then indicates using their eye movements when the correct letter is presented. Letter by letter the person is then able to spell out words to the communication partner. An example is shown below. The communication partner points at the A and asks the patient if their letter is in the first row. If the patient communicates 'yes' (by looking up) then the partner goes through the row letter by letter until they reach the right answer, i.e. if the patient indicates 'yes' their letter is A, then the communication partner writes this down and asks the patient to think of the next letter of their word, whereas if the patient indicates 'no' (by holding their gaze level or looking down), the partner checks whether it is B, C, or D in turn. If the patient's initial response was that their letter was not in the first row, the partner moves down the vowels column until the patient indicates that they have reached the row in which their letter can be found.

A	B	C	D		
E	F	G	H		
I	J	K	L	M	N
O	P	Q	R	S	T
U	V	W	X	Y	Z

It is important to remember that setting the person up for a conversation can take time (positioning, hoisting, suctioning, respirators, getting the aid in the right place, etc) and letter by letter spelling is much slower than speech. It is our experience that there will be people with LIS who use the communication aids in a similar way to texting and will use abbreviations (such as 'L8R'), or be willing for the communication partner to make guesses at what they are trying to say (such as 'you have spelt N-E-U-R-O-P-S-Y are you wanting to say neuropsychologist?') which can speed up communication and reduce effort for the person with LIS. Indeed, higher-tech aids such as computerised eye gaze systems often include predictive text options, and patients who can learn to use these aids proficiently can often select their target word after one or two letters if it is a high-frequency word. However, we regularly see people with LIS who do indeed want to state everything in full themselves and decline the option of guessing from their communication partner, however laborious it is for them and the partner. At times people may also withdraw from a contact by closing their eyes and keeping them closed or not moving their eyes at all, and this may be the only way a person can signal they have had enough and do not want to continue.

It is important to keep the person's individual needs at the centre of any interaction. Critical to neurorehabilitation is an understanding of the very effortful nature for the person with LIS using their eye movements to communicate and asking staff to participate in experiential learning with each other in training sessions can help with this. When asking staff to practice communicating 'yes' and 'no' only using eye movements, we encourage them to reflect on how it feels when you want to say 'yes, *but…*' or 'yes…*and…*' but communication and the way a question has been phrased doesn't allow for it. When asking staff to try spelling words letter by letter with a communication partner, we encourage them to reflect on the time and effort it takes, but also how it could feel to be communicating about one's innermost thoughts and challenging feelings using this method, and how the communication partner can make assumptions about broader meaning when the sentences are brief (reading between the lines) that may be erroneous or distracting. This can really help develop a richer understanding and give first-hand experience of the potential need for shorter sessions, the speed and number of clinical tasks you will be able to accomplish in sessions, and the need to provide breaks to rest the eyes. It is key to not assume the person with LIS will have self-awareness and insight into their increasing fatigue, so learning what to watch for when working with someone communicating this way is important to prompt the clinician to provide opportunities for rest, and/or to end the session with the aim of continuing at another time. We encourage staff to reflect on if you only had short periods of the day when you can do this, who would you really want to use your communication energy with? It is critical to balance the opportunities and time for clinical communication with the patient's wider recreational, social, and emotional needs. Patients who can learn to use eye gaze may be able to access environmental controls, email, and the internet and may prefer to prioritise leisure activities above clinical assessments; agreeing on a balance that suits them is therefore important.

Within supervision sessions, it is helpful to reflect on the direction of conversation and who has the power in this. Being dependent on others to initiate conversation is deeply frustrating for many, and then trying to steer the conversation to a new topic when your conversation partner has a session plan that they are following can result in a withdrawal from communication and have a negative impact on mood. There is a skill in starting from a very wide conversation starter and honing it to the topic a person wants to discuss without exhausting them, and learning this skill requires some careful reflection and practice for those of us who work with this group of people.

Given sessions are often shorter and require the clinician to be active in recording letter by letter what the person is communicating, session planning is essential. The clinician can find it hard to mentally hold in working memory everything that is being spelled out and having a whiteboard visible to both you and the person with LIS to reduce these demands on you both can be helpful. With the patient's consent, it can be helpful to have a third person such as an assistant present to write the responses on the whiteboard, whilst the clinician keeps their focus on the patient. You do not want to be wasting too much time of the critical window when the person is optimised to use the aids. You will need to have a clear session plan perhaps with periods of closed questions to speed up communication before asking open ended questions. Thought to counter balancing questions and checking answers is important, particularly if the answer appears impossible, for example, if the patient begins to spell a combination of letters that cannot lead to a word (e.g. 'STPC'), or if it is unclear whether they have completed the word and moved onto the next one (e.g. 'THE' may be a complete word, or may be the start of a longer word such as 'THERE', 'THEIR', 'THEMATIC'). Patients may make spelling errors, particularly if they had limited education or specific learning difficulties such as dyslexia prior to injury; for these patients, facilitating them to spell a longer string of letters may then help the clinician decipher the meaning.

It is also important to be aware that patients may use different communication systems at different times. A patient who can use eye gaze during the day, when they are fully awake and alert, can be positioned comfortably in their wheelchair, and their eye gaze equipment can be set up and calibrated optimally. They are not going to be able to use the same method of communication when they are tired in bed, when positioning the equipment effectively is likely to be challenging. Using alternative methods at such times, such as closed questions or an alphabet chart, is likely to be needed. Involving patients as co-authors of their guidelines for such circumstances is recommended, as they can help identify the most efficient ways of asking key questions and feel a sense of autonomy at being actively involved.

For those who can learn to use higher technological communication options, like the ability to access email, this can open opportunities for session design, such as sending an agenda in advance with some prepared questions the person can respond to in their own time to show you when you meet.

Working with people with LIS requires flexibility, personalization, and creativity. One of the authors has facilitated a psychological resilience and coping group of five people with LIS who were parents but living away from their families in a residential care service. All group members were able to use email. The group agreed a series of themes for the group sessions to focus on. All group members were sent a series of questions to consider and pre-pare answers to for sharing at the next group meeting. In this way the group could share with each other when they came together using the text-to-talk option on their device. This enabled other group members to listen to their views, and the members could share with each other their own thoughts and feelings about parenting with LIS whilst living away from the family home. As a peer group, they were able to provide ideas for each other about how to remain engaged in family life, places that worked for them to visit as a family, and ideas for how to spend time in the service when family were visiting. It created a therapeutic space for normalisation, shared problem solving, resili-ence, and hope building.

It is not uncommon, in our experience with people with LIS, that once their physical world is dramatically curtailed by the injury, they often develop a large online world. Technology advances such as video calling, text to voice software, and eye control computer interfaces enable people with LIS to both maintain and develop their personal networks. For some, this has enabled periods of creative productivity involving writing, drawing, and music making. Perhaps most well-known is Jean-Dominique Bauby's memoir, The Diving Bell and the Butterfly (although this was dictated using a low tech, alphabet board), but we have also worked with patients who have used high-tech aids to write poetry or music, construct DJ-sets and write presentations that they have then delivered to an audience of professionals via the voice output on their AAC device. A recent book collated by Keen (2025) shares an inter-national and personal perspective of people living with locked-in syndrome.

Returning to some of the key themes in working with people with severe brain injury, once a form of communication is established, this enables the opportunity to assess cognition, psychological state, and any behavioural issues of concern. These are considered in turn below.

9.1 Cognition

Once a method of reliable communication has been achieved, in-depth assessment of cognition can occur. Whilst in Classic LIS, it is understood that there is cortical sparing of the higher order functions, and there are several reasons why cognitive assessment can be needed. Firstly, as described earlier in this chapter, misdiagnosis is possible as both under- and over-estimates of cognition can occur (Laureys et al., 2005; Crawford et al., 2023). Obviously, correctly identifying if a person is in LIS with largely intact cognition is important as all decisions about their life, future, and day-to-day care and existence are theirs to make, even though they are physically dependent on others. Supporting such people to manage change and adjust to a new way of living where their 'voice' is central to care planning, and decision-making is vital. At other times, the reverse is possible, when the person may be assumed to be in LIS but actually is *less* cognitively able and instead has gross physical or sensory impairments and cognitive impairments or is actually in PDOC with roving eye movements. There is also the possibility that patients who present with the tetraplegia and anarthria typical of LIS may have a more complex cognitive picture, in which they can make some capacitous decisions but not others. The literature does report people with LIS who have experienced some cognitive changes (Schnakers et al., 2008; Rousseaux et al., 2009; Trojano et al., 2010; Wilson et al., 2011). Systematic neuropsychological assessment is needed to establish rehabilitation and communication optimisation (Rousseaux et al., 2009).

Obviously, given the severe disability encompassing speech and movement (limiting positioning and energy levels, etc), people with LIS are complex to assess. Many standardised neuropsychological assessment tools may be unsuitable for use or may require some adaptations (Wilson et al., 2011). Several studies have described cognitive assessments of people with LIS, outlining which assessment tools can be used, which either rely on binary responses, forced choices, or short-answer responses (which can be answered using letter-by-letter spelling), and some of these are displayed below to demonstrate examples that readers may wish to consider using. However, we recommend following the approach outlined in Crawford et al. (2023) in which an individual formulation-driven assessment is designed that is focussed on answering key clinical questions and determination of focal versus global deficits, as opposed to a 'LIS battery' approach and administration of all the possible tests that could be used.

Domain	Allain et al. (1998)	Schnakers et al. (2008)	Wilson et al. (2011)	Marino et al. (2018)	Crawford et al. (2023)
Premorbid functioning			Spot the Word		Spot the Wordv2
General cognitive abilities	Ravens coloured progressive matrices		Matrix Reasoning (WAIS-IV)	Ravens progressive matrices	Matrix Reasoning (WAIS-IV)
Basic Visuoperceptual abilities				BORB	VOSP
Verbal and Language abilities	Verbal WAIS-R subtests Verbal Comprehension BDAE Written Comprehension BDAE	Word-Picture Naming Picture Vocabulary test		Linguistic comprehension Test (AAT)	Functional assessment of spelling in communication
Memory abilities	Digit Span (forwards and backwards) WAIS-R Rey 15 words Paired associatesWMS-R Delayed Recognition BEM 144	Doors	Face and Picture Recognition RBMT-3 CVLT	Verbal memory test with visual cue (TEMA)	Three picture Pyramids and Palm Trees test Face and Picture Recognition RBMT-3 Camden Memory Test for Words Doors

Attentional abilities		Bespoke auditory attention task			
Executive functioning abilities	Largely intact cognitive functioning	Shortened WCST		WCST	Brixton
Findings	Largely intact cognitive functioning	Largely intact cognitive functioning Impairments related to organic damage beyond brainstem	Largely intact cognitive functioning Impairments secondary to sensory changes (diplopia and blurred vision)	Largely intact cognitive functioning Weaker executive functioning and verbal memory	Cases were illustrative of different levels of cognitive impairment

Notes: AAT: Aachener Aphasie Test; BDAE: Boston Diagnostic Aphasia Examination; BEM: Batterie d'efficience mnesique; BORB: Birmingham Object Recognition Battery; Brixton: Hayling and Brixton Test; CVLT: California Verbal Learning Test; Doors: Doors and People Test; RBMT-3: Rivermead Behavioural Memory Test-Third Edition; TEMA: Test di Memoria e Apprendimento; VOSP: Visual Object Spatial Perception Battery; WAIS-R: Wechsler Adult Intelligence Scale-Revised; WAIS-IV: Wechsler Adult Intelligence Scale-Fourth Edition; WMS-R: Wechsler Memory Scale-Revised; WCST: Wisconsin Card Sorting Test.

Whilst the tests outlined above will typically be administered by a psychologist, other formal and informal assessments relevant to understanding the person's cognition will be carried out by other members of the team, particularly SLT and OT. Informal observations of how easily the patient learns to use communication aids, how effectively they use them across settings, and how flexible or rigid they are in sessions will all inform understanding. All clinicians will share their assessment findings with the aim of creating a shared formulation of the person's abilities. These discussions often require the need to carefully address principles of psychometric assessment and differentiate between here and now concrete decision making versus abstract reasoning and thought. Once a person's abilities are thoroughly understood, advocacy to ensure that their rights to decision-making and consent to care and treatment is important. Feedback and psychoeducation for both the patient themselves and their wider family and friends are also vital in order that they also understand the cognitive profile, have clarity about the person's abilities, and that they are supported to maximise their interactions together. Issues around supporting mental capacity and working with families are outlined in more detail later in this chapter.

9.2 Emotion and psychological functioning

Due to the person's movement impairment, they are unable to show any facial expression. This blank and flat affect means they are unable to convey their internal emotional state (such as not being able to look sad, happy, angry, or fearful). It is not uncommon to be working with someone who suddenly starts sobbing, in floods of tears and overwhelmed by their emotion but with this occurring entirely silently as they are unable to produce any sound (anarthia). Or, to be working with someone who is very angry and spelling out, with your support, their significant frustrations and annoyance, yet their face has not been able to alter, remains blank, and cannot reflect this strong emotion. In addition, this blank facial affect creates challenges for clinicians as the typical cues that we rely upon to evaluate and determine our therapeutic rapport and validations, as therapists are absent. It is necessary to be more overt and direct in talking with people with LIS about the value of sessions for them. The challenges this presents for clinicians can be illustrated by a reflection from a trainee who was supervised by one of the authors when working with 'Tim' (a pseudonym):

> "Working with someone who cannot talk and was not able to form facial expressions was certainly a learning experience for me in how I judge whether rapport is built, if I have engaged a client and how successful our therapy is".

Tim wanted to learn about LIS and they spent time learning about other people's experiences and looking at information about LIS. The trainee reflected:

> *"I found myself constantly doubting myself professionally and person-ally and questioning the utility of our sessions, purely because I was not getting any verbal or non-verbal feedback from Tim and he declined to use low- and high-tech communication systems in sessions…It was not until we were nearing the end of our sessions that I began to recognise the contribution of our sessions in his rehabilitation; Tim's parents gave glowing feedback and knowing he wished to continue learning about others' experiences showed me that he had found our sessions helpful. How ironic that it was not until I had verbal feedback from his parents that I started feeling validated!"*

This inability to create any facial expression can lead to misattributions about the person's internal experiences, such as assumptions about the person having low mood and poor quality of life in the context of so much dis-ability. We encourage staff to examine their own preconceptions and beliefs about severe neuro-disability. The so-called 'disability paradox' is helpful to consider.

> *Why do many people with serious and persistent disabilities report that they experience a good or excellent quality of life when to most external observers these people seem to live an undesirable daily existence?*
>
> (Albrecht & Devlieger, 1999)

People with LIS do live with dramatic and massive changes in their abilities, independence and lifestyle. Despite the predictions and expectations of their family and many clinicians, research indicates that self-reported mood states and quality of life can be good (Lulé et al., 2009) with the majority of low quality of life scores stemming from motor impairments (Halan et al., 2021). In people with longstanding LIS, most endorsed being 'happy' which correlated with the length of time since their diagnosis (Bruno et al., 2011) and successful psychological adjustment to LIS related to problem-oriented coping strategies, like seeking information and emotional coping strategies (Lule et al., 2009). In countries where euthanasia is permitted, the demand for this from people with LIS has been described as 'surprisingly low' (Laureys et al., 2005).

This is something that we have experienced firsthand in working with people with LIS. For example, a person who acquired LIS following a stroke who wanted to discuss an advanced directive for his care. He began the con-versation by asking if it would be possible for his life to be ended. Given the effort involved in communication, his question was blunt and not surrounded by any reasoning or explanation. Assumptions were made about this question, and his family was very distressed. However, the question was not a request to end his life but about finding the facts of what was and was not possible. A detailed piece of work was done over a period of several sessions in which the patient and one of the authors first identified the reasons for this question and some of his following questions. This highlighted that he was dealing with his adjustment to his profound disability and felt that he was able to manage his physical and communicative limitations, as long as he did not lose what he referred to as his intellectual capability. The nub of his questions was about the likelihood and consequences of any further strokes and whether he could refuse treatment if, in addition to his current disability, he became cognitively impaired. This frank discussion, achieved through the use of an alphabet chart, enabled a careful plan of questions that he wanted to discuss with his consultant in rehabilitation medicine and ultimately an advance directive being made about what treatment he would and would not accept if he were to become ill. He expressed a clear wish to be treated for all conditions unless they were to lead to a permanent reduction in his cognitive functioning. This was a very different conversation than had first been envisaged when he asked his question about ending his own life, and it highlights the importance of taking the time to find out the full question in a context where a person may not provide a great deal of detail. It also highlighted the importance of providing a full answer with all the detail then required for a person to reach a considered and informed decision about matters of such great importance.

Nonetheless, some studies have indicated that a minority of people with LIS (around one-third of the study population) reported being 'unhappy' (Bruno et al., 2011), and depression (mild-moderate) has been reported to be more common in people with LIS than in the general population (Halan et al., 2021). These contrasting findings show that individualised assessment and formulation are needed.

Other emotion-related phenomena such as pathological laughing and crying have been reported in people with LIS that was not related to a mood disorder and did not improve with pharmacological treatment (Sacco et al., 2008). The study authors hypothesised that this was the result of the brain lesion extending into the ponto-cerebellar pathway.

When concerns about mood and emotions are being raised about people with LIS, clinicians are encouraged to examine why these concerns are being highlighted, given the potential for fundamental misattributions about a person's internal mood state being due to their lack of facial expression and the assumptions others make about how people 'must' feel with that severity of disability.

Any assessment of mood and emotion must be guided by the person's communication and cognitive abilities. For example, the method of com-munication (can you ask open questions or must you use closed questions?), whether the person has the working memory abilities to answer standardised questionnaires (which typically involve holding up to four options in mind when answering a question), how quickly they fatigue, and the severity of their neuro-disability which requires reliance on others (for set up seating, positioning, hoisting, suctioning, etc). Clearly asking a person about an internal emotional state requires a level of cognition (see Chapter 6), and many standardised questionnaires are not suitable for clinical populations with severe cognitive impairments (Rose et al., 2022). Caution is needed in making extrapolations from responses a person may give, especially when these are binary questions (see Chapter 4). If open questions are not possible, then selection of an image to convey an underlying emotion (emoji faces, line drawings, Likert scales, etc.) may be tried although it is important to check the person's ability to identify these emotions before assuming that they might be able to relate them to their own internal mood state. Whilst these are suggestions for how mood and emotion might be assessed directly with patients in LIS, thought should be given as to whether formal measures are needed at all and for what purpose. Patients rarely perceive changes on questionnaire scores to be of personal value, and the clinical focus may be more usefully applied to exploring any factors that support their well-being and quality of life and how to promote these.

Typically in clinical practice, a multifactorial approach to assessment of mood, emotion, and well-being will be needed, combining direct assessment findings with other information such as your own direct observations of the patient, observations reported by others, and monitoring of records that detail the range of activities and responses a person has made, in order to arrive at a formulation of any presenting difficulties. The patient should be supported to generate ideas for how they believe any difficulties could be improved. Psychological therapy can be aimed at improving mood, resilience, adjustment to disability, self-advocacy, well-being, and coping but must be tailored according to the person's cognitive impairments. In our experience, practical-supported problem solving and ensuring the person's 'voice', values, and wishes are expressed in the care plan is a core part of working with people in the early stages. The clinician should therefore be open-minded to the idea that their main role might be to advocate for the patient around factors such as how to improve their physical discomfort, how to help staff communicate with them more effectively, or how to access more quality time (remotely or in person) with their family, rather than on talking therapies or other psychological interventions. Nevertheless, in our experience, patients in LIS can gain considerable benefit from psychological support to help them contextualise and normalise their experiences and think about some of the more challenging aspects of their disability. We have found that using resources such as newspaper articles, videos, and social media featuring other people with LIS can be enormously helpful to patients. Some patients wish to hear only positive, hopeful stories, whereas other patients have wanted to hear about a wider range of experiences, including those where other people with LIS have reported frustration, hopelessness or even explored assisted dying. The important factors for the clinician to be aware of are to support the patient to be in control of what resources are accessed and to have the skills to help them manage any emotional reactions and reflect on the materials they have viewed and the impact on them. Some patients choose to access these resources with family present, e.g. one of our patients chose to watch the film of The Diving Bell and the Butterfly with a close relative, and used this experience to communicate which aspects of the story resonated with him and why, helping the relative to gain a broader understanding of his adjustment to his condition.

9.3 Behaviour

In our experience, the behaviour of some people with LIS can be seen by staff as challenging and difficult, often when they are exerting great and pedantic levels of control and rigidity over how they communicate with staff and how their care is delivered or other aspects of their environments. Our experience is that this type of behaviour is often interpreted by staff as attributable to the patient's premorbid 'personality' or psychological 'adjustment' issues, and these behaviours are presented to neuropsychologists and neuropsychiatrists by the wider team as something needing urgent resolution. It is important to highlight that people with LIS have little body autonomy and personal control and have often had experience of being talked about like an object whilst they are present in the room. It can also be challenging to ensure that all care staff, including agency staff, have been adequately trained to use patients' preferred communication methods, and staff may be under too much time pressure to work through a flowchart of the person's needs. These factors can lead to patients feeling frustrated and upset and even keener to persist with getting their specific message across. Cognitive factors may also play a role, and we have speculated elsewhere about why difficulties with executive functioning may occur in this patient group due to factors such as organic damage beyond the brainstem and/or a possible 'use it or lose it' phenomenon in people who have so few opportunities for everyday problem-solving due to their physical disabilities (Crawford et al., 2023). Developing a nuanced understanding of the person's rigidity and inflexibility in relation to their environment stemming from formulating loss of control and/or consideration to cognitive factors for rigidity of thought and/or premorbid factors is needed. However, management strategies may be similar regardless of the underlying cause, including empowering patients to write their own guidelines, and, where possible, to be directly involved in training staff in how to implement these and working with staff teams to support their understanding of the formulation, address fundamental attribution errors, and develop their understanding of the person's situation, e.g. through experiential learning as described earlier in this chapter.

It is also apparent that for people with LIS who reside in hospital and residential care facilities, it can be difficult for staff to be given time to spend with them for general conversation beyond care tasks, particularly given their slow speed of communication. This can greatly limit the number and quality of interaction opportunities a person with LIS has. In addition to their wider networks of family and friends, it can be invaluable to explore the use of trained volunteers to act as communication partners and personal assistants for leisure activities and conversation.

9.4 Mental capacity

As has been outlined earlier in this chapter, if a person with LIS has broadly intact cognition, then they are likely to have the mental capacity to make all decisions for themselves, including complex decisions. Indeed, for these patients, the first principle of the MCA, the presumption of capacity, is likely to apply. However, it is vital that patients are given appropriate support to make their own informed decisions, including ensuring that they are provided with all of the information pertinent to the decision and that they are given opportunities to ask questions, seek further information, and have time to consider their decision. They will also need their communication aids set up optimally, at a time of day when they are fully awake and alert, in order to communicate their decisions. They thus need skilled support to exercise their autonomy, although this support should be conceptualised as support for their physical and communication difficulties, rather than as support to pass the functional test of capacity.

When patients in LIS have more extensive cognitive impairments, any capacity assessment requires careful planning in advance in order to maximise the patient's ability to demonstrate capacity if they are able. Thought should be given to how to present the pertinent information, constructing balanced closed questions around understanding and retention of the information in advance of sessions, and how to phrase questions that assess the patient's ability to use and weigh the information. The latter is ideally assessed via open questions, although closed questions can be constructed where pros and cons/risks and benefits to the patient are known.

It should be noted that the MCA Code of Practice (2007) specifically mentions LIS in Section 4.23, in which it states that

> *Sometimes there is no way for a person to communicate. This will apply to very few people, but it does include:*
>
> * *people who are unconscious or in a coma, or*
> * *those with the very rare condition sometimes known as 'locked-in syndrome', who are conscious but cannot speak or move at all.*
>
> *If a person cannot communicate their decision in any way at all, the Act says they should be treated as if they are unable to make that decision.*

As can be seen from the quote above, there is an assumption that people with LIS cannot communicate; however, this is not the case for the majority of these patients, only those who present with tetraplegia, anarthria and PDOC.

We would therefore emphasise the importance of determining communication methods for people with LIS and giving them all necessary support to make their own decisions wherever possible.

9.5 Working with families

The experience of seeing someone they love have a severe brain injury such that they present with the profound physical disabilities of locked in syndrome can be devastating for families. This chapter has made some references to how families can be included in therapeutic work with the patient and with the patient's consent. However, families may also benefit from psychological support to explore factors such as their own reactions to the situation, including emotions such as loss and anger, anxieties around the practical implications of the changes the person with LIS has experienced and problem-solving challenges around planning for the future. Psychoeducation for both adults and children may be helpful, not just around the disabilities and limitations but also the strengths of the person with LIS, the range of activities they can still do, and how they can have quality interactions as a family. Techniques for working with families are outlined in more detail in Chapter 10.

9.6 Summary

In summary, people with LIS present with a range of difficulties requiring support from skilled clinicians. The importance of working as a team is vital, with both distinct and overlapping roles between different disciplines. We have focused primarily on the areas of most relevance to psychology, but the most powerful interventions for emotion and well-being in this patient group may often be around medical and other aspects of physical care, specialist communication support, and promoting good systemic working such as a shared team formulation and commitment to empowering patients to direct their own care and make their own decisions. Nevertheless, psychologists have important roles to play in understanding the barriers to communication, assessing cognition, emotional functioning, and behaviour, and providing person-centred interventions to both patients and their families.

References

Albrecht, G. L., & Devlieger, P. J. (1999). The disability paradox: High quality of life against all odds. *Social Science & Medicine, 48*(8), 977–988.

Allain, P., Joseph, P. A., Isambert, J. L., Le Gall, D., & Emile J. (1998). Cognitive functions in chronic locked-in syndrome: A report of two cases. *Cortex, 34*, 629–634.

Bauer, G., Gerstenbrand, F., & Rumpl, E. (1979). Varieties of the locked-in syndrome. *Journal of Neurology, 221*(2), 77–91.

Bruno, M. A., Schnakers, C., Damas, F., Pellas, F., Lutte, I., Bernheim, J., Majerus, S., Moonen, G., Goldman, S., & Laureys, S. (2009). Locked-in syndrome in children: Report of five cases and review of the literature. *Pediatric Neurology, 41*(4), 237–246.

Bruno, M. A., Vanhaudenhuyse, A., Thibaut, A., Moonen, G., & Laureys, S. (2011). From unresponsive wakefulness to minimally conscious PLUS and functional locked-in syndromes: Recent advances in our understanding of disorders of consciousness. *Journal of Neurology*, 258(7), 1373–1384.

Casanova, E., Lazzari, R. E., Lotta, S., & Mazzucchi, A. (2003). Locked-in syndrome: Improvement in the prognosis after an early intensive multidisciplinary rehabilitation. *Archives of Physical Medicine and Rehabilitation, 84*(6), 862–867.

Crawford, S., Connolly, S. & Rose, A. E. (2023) The importance of accuracy when diagnosing locked in syndrome (p 316–361). In Fish, J., Betteridge, S., & Wilson, B.A. (Eds.). Rare Conditions, Diagnostic Challenges, and Controversies in Clinical Neuropsychology: Out of the Ordinary (1st ed.). Routledge.

Das, J. M., Anosike, K., & Asuncion, R. M. D. (2023). Locked-in syndrome. In: *StatPearls*. StatPearls Publishing.

Halan, T., Ortiz, J. F., Reddy, D., Altamimi, A., Ajibowo, A. O., & Fabara, S. P. (2021). Locked-in syndrome: A systematic review of long-term management and prognosis. *Cureus, 13*(7), e16727.

Hocker, S., & Wijdicks, E. F. M. (2015) Recovery from locked-in syndrome. *JAMA Neurology, 72*(7):832–833. https://doi.org/0.1001/jamaneurol.2015.0479

Keen, S. (Ed.). (2025). *Giving a voice to those living with locked-in syndrome: Sharing feelings, experiences, hopes and expectations.* Routledge.

Laureys, S., Pellas, F., Van Eeckhout, P., Ghorbel, S., Schnakers, C., Perrin, F., Berré, J., Faymonville, M. E., Pantke, K. H., Damas, F., Lamy, M., Moonen, G., & Goldman, S. (2005). The locked-in syndrome: What is it like to be conscious but paralyzed and voiceless?. *Progress in Brain Research, 150*, 495–511.

Lugo, Z., Bruno, M-A., Gosseries, O., Demertizi, A., Heine, L., Thonnard, M., Blandin, V., Pellas, F & Laureys, S. (2015). Beyond the gaze: Communicating in chronic locked-in syndrome. *Brain Injury, 29*, 1056–1061.

Lulé, D., Zickler, C., Häcker, S., Bruno, M. A., Demertzi, A., Pellas, F., Laureys, S., & Kübler, A. (2009). Life can be worth living in locked-in syndrome. *Progress in Brain Research, 177*, 339–351.

Marino, S., Corallo, F., Allone, C., Formica, C., Alagna, A., Todaro, A., Pollicino, P., Rifici, C., & Sessa, E. (2018). Clinical and neurocognitive outcome evaluation in locked-in syndrome. *Biomedical Journal of Scientific & Technical Research, 12*(1), 8999–9003.

Nilsen, H. W., Martinsen, A. C. T., Johansen, I., Kirkevold, M., Sunnerhagen, S. & Becker, F. (2023). Demographic, medical, and clinical characteristics of a population-based sample of patients with long-lasting locked-in syndrome. *Neurology*, 101 (10). https://doi.org/10.1212/WNL.0000000000207577

Office of the Public Guardian (2007). Mental Capacity Act Code of Practice. www.gov.uk/government/publications/mental-capacity-act-code-of-practice.

Patterson, J. R., & Grabois, M. (1986). Locked-in syndrome: a review of 139 cases. *Stroke, 17*(4), 758–764

Rose, A., Cullen, B., Crawford, S., & Evans, J. J. (2022). A systematic review of mood and depression measures in people with severe cognitive and communication impairments following acquired brain injury. *Clinical Rehabilitation*, 37(5), 679–700. https://doi.org/10.1177/02692155221139023

Rousseaux, M., Castelnot, E., Rigaux, P., Kozlowski, O., & Danzé, F. (2009). Evidence of persisting cognitive impairment in a case series of patients with locked-in syndrome. *Journal of Neurology, Neurosurgery, and Psychiatry, 80*(2), 166–170.

Sacco, S., Sarà, M., Pistoia, F., Conson, M., Albertini, G., & Carolei, A. (2008). Management of pathologic laughter and crying in patients with locked-in syndrome: A report of 4 cases. *Archives of Physical Medicine and Rehabilitation, 89*(4), 775–778.

Schnakers, C., Majerus, S., Goldman, S., Boly, M., Van Eeckhout, P., Gay, S., Pellas, F., Bartsch, V., Peigneux, P., Moonen, G., & Laureys, S. (2008). Cognitive function in the locked-in syndrome. *Journal of Neurology, 255*(3), 323–330.

Schnakers, C., Perrin, F., Schabus, M., Hustinx, R., Majerus, S., Moonen, G., Boly, M., Vanhaudenhuyse, M. A. & Laureys, S. (2009). Detecting consciousness in a total locked-in syndrome: An active event-related paradigm. *Neurocase, 15*, 271–277.

Schnetzer, L., McCoy, M., Bergmann, J., Kunz, A., Leis, S., & Trinka, E. (2023). Locked-in syndrome revisited. *Therapeutic Advances in Neurological Disorders, 16*, 17562864231160873. https://doi.org/10.1177/17562864231160873

Smith, E., & Delargy, M. (2005). Locked-in syndrome. *BMJ (Clinical research ed.), 330*(7488), 406–409

Trojano, L., Moretta, P., Estraneo, A., & Santoro, L. (2010). Neuropsychologic assessment and cognitive rehabilitation in a patient with locked-in syndrome and left neglect. *Archives of Physical Medicine and Rehabilitation, 91*(3), 498–502.

Wilson, B. A., Hinchcliffe, A., Okines, T., Florschutz, G., & Fish, J. (2011). A case study of locked-in-syndrome: Psychological and personal perspectives. *Brain Injury, 25*(5), 526–538.

Yokose, M., Furuya, K., Suzuki, M., Ozawa, T., Kim, Y., Miura, K., Matsuzono, K., Mashiko, T., Tada, M., Koide, R., Shimazaki, H., Matsuura, T., & Fujimoto, S. (2018). Vertical gaze palsy caused by selective unilateral rostral midbrain infarction. *Neuro-ophthalmology, 42*(5), 309–311.

10 Working with families in complex neuro-disability

That car didn't just crash into him, it smashed into and ran over all of our lives. We have all been changed forever

(Wife of a man in a PDOC)

It is often said that whilst the brain injury has happened to one person, all the people in their wider networks are also impacted. It is inevitable that these networks have unique, complex histories, and family dynamics (Smith & Worthington, 2024). We use the word 'families' in this chapter to mean those naturalistic support networks formed by those closest to the person (biological, legal, or family of choice and selection). It is important that staff are mindful of cultural factors that are relevant to understanding that person as an individual, such as being aware that in many African cultures, the use of familial descriptors such as Auntie or Sister do not necessarily refer to a biological family member; and that many immigrants may not have biological family in their adopted home and instead have selected and built a family of choice around their life. Staff will need to work hard to identify who is in the network and who may be excluded and why. Cultural factors will also influence family members' perspectives of 'illness' and 'disability', and understanding this is important when dealing with and appreciating incomplete recovery and ongoing disability (Klonoff et al., 2017). For most people in the family, the injury is their first encounter of severe brain damage, and their first experience of beginning to consider how brains work, how brains get hurt, and who and what helps people to recover. The family is thrust onto a roller coaster of learning.

Western approaches to neurorehabilitation have a tendency to focus on the individual, albeit with acknowledgement of the wider family, but legal and policy requirements limit information sharing (confidentiality) and access (hospital visiting hours) and proxy decision-making when the person cannot make decisions for themselves (mental capacity). This approach to neurorehabilitation may be an anathema to some families for whom care should be provided substantively by family and who may hold cultural views

DOI: 10.4324/9781032665986-10

about the appropriateness of professional carers such as those of a different gender attending to someone in their family. Whilst some families will be keen for the clinical staff to lead and guide, others will want to do their own research and reading. Many will feel dissatisfied with the apparent slow speed of assessment processes (hypotheses generation, testing, and iterative refinement over time) and recovery trajectories in severe brain injury, compared to assessment and treatment in other medical domains. They may have really lost trust and faith in healthcare professionals as the journey through acute and post-acute services has progressed. Here, the internet can be both helpful and unhelpful. Complex neuro-disability is multi-factorial and difficult to wrangle, even for experienced clinicians in the field. The challenge for families to navigate through the volume of internet provision to determine which information is similar to their situation and of any quality is difficult. It is likely that families' differing views about medicine, healing, and well-being will also become more obvious. Some families will want alternative and complementary therapies tried, and just as the evidence base in this population is challenging for traditional neurorehabilitation, it is certainly the case in alternative approaches. We have discovered families dropping various essential oils in PEGs and blocking these, or sneaking in craniosacral therapists when the person does not have intact skull bones etc. Working with the family to look at their suggestions and be clear on who their suggestion is really for and what can be trialled safely is important (for example, Reiki may be fine but acupuncture may not be). Decision-making about which approaches can be safely trialled and what assurances are required from any outside practitioners is needed. How families respond to trying to navigate these potential restrictions on what they see would be right or best for the person can be informative in understanding their own personal formulations of the issues, their active or avoidant coping styles and the wider family dynamics that will need to be worked within.

Complex neuro-disability creates information vacuums. The person themselves is rarely able to communicate or recall information to share with their family about what they have been doing and key details about their day or progress. Visitors often seek out staff to ask for information about the person and try to gain a sense of their days and a sense of continuity. It is of interest that in other settings such as childcare or doggy daycare, it is common for the family to receive several photos and updates of the activities that their cherished family member has been doing and a handover at the end of the day. This helps with maintaining and continuing bonds between the network and enabling a sense of shared understanding. However, any equivalence of this is rarely done in busy western health settings. Instead, there is a concept of a 'Family Meeting' where several days or weeks into admissions, the family has access to the team to hear about assessments and goals, but that day-to-day experience of the person is rarely captured and shared.

Often well-intentioned attempts to protect children from the realities of the injury leave them in their own unique information vacuum. Clearly, seeing someone who you love with significant parts of their skull removed, in wheelchairs, hospital gowns, with pipes and tubes, making strange sounds or not acknowledging you at all is deeply painful for children and indeed all the family. Equally, being kept away from the person, not being able to see them and witnessing the distress of others is frightening and scary too. For families trying to negotiate how to support the children of a profoundly injured parent, great amounts of fear develop about determining what is best to do. It is important that children are not forgotten by professionals and that the family is facilitated to think about the child's needs, age and developmental stage, how to best answer questions and model interactions with the injured parent. Children typically are not able to source a peer network and connect with other children of people with such profound injuries. We have often met younger children who have done their own secret internet searches and been distressed by imagining what their parent was like, as well as very young children who happily climb on the bed and snuggle up to a parent who is unaware of their presence. Adult inpatient hospital settings by their nature are often some distance from the family home, will have a great many other profoundly brain-injured patients who can be frightening for children, and these settings invariably don't cater to the needs of children. Developing a special selection of things for visiting that they can do (such as make a music playlist to play) or a special toy that they can play with there may be helpful. The team may be supportive in developing activities for children who get bored at the bedside, and the wider family, built on observations during personalised assessments. Any emotion-related behaviours that are typically associated with pleasure, and also any activities that are particularly helpful to families (for example, to push the wheelchair on a walk outside, or showing off their football skills on the grounds, reading to the person, or rubbing hand cream into their skin) are important to incorporate whether or not the patient shows signs of recognition or pleasure, provided that there are no signs of distress.

The needs of the family carers of the person should always be considered by the clinical teams, despite families' common reluctance for this (such as feeling 'I will focus on myself when he is better'). Research has repeatedly illustrated clinical levels of psychological distress, carer burden and strain, compassion fatigue, social isolation, and/or role changes in families of people with brain injuries. Given the entire family system is disrupted by the injury, as time progresses from the bedside vigil and acute survival issues to longer term post-acute assessment and neurorehabilitation, the alterations in roles, finances, and demands of real life (work, childcare, mortgages etc) need focus. The Care Act (2014) in England and Wales sets out a legal responsibility on the Local Authority to ensure that the needs of carers are considered and met. Often there will be a social worker in the service who will lead on thinking with families about their own needs, but responsibility can also be on any member of the team acting as the patient's key worker who has regular contact with family members and routinely this will involve a psychologist. We are often asked whether family members who do not themselves have a brain injury really require therapeutic interventions from a neuropsychologist. The short answer is, not necessarily. However, in our experience, for some families, it is necessary to have a clinical neuropsychologist present who is well versed in the diagnostic issues, rehabilitation intricacies, the realistic prognosis for complex neuro-disability, and the common themes that families face with this in their lives. It is not uncommon to hear families have been advised to maintain unrealistic levels of hope, or that they should just focus on themselves first, or that the person with the brain injury should be told how their behaviour is impacting the family member and take some responsibility for it. This has hampered family members' sense-making and formulation about the nature and impact of the brain injury. Whoever the source of support, the emphasis should be on emotional support, enhancing self-care, education, and sense-making.

Families often talk about the challenges of keeping others informed about progress, finding time for their own self-care, the challenges of financial costs associated with loss of income/travelling to be at the hospital and the sadness associated with being at home alone. We have seen various practical strategies help the person's networks such as:

- appointing a social media update lead to provide agreed information to a wider group and decrease the reliance on the key family members to do this (daily, several times a week, weekly, monthly, etc);
- online rotas of friends and family who help with childcare responsibilities, meal provision, and grocery shopping
- online rotas for visiting the person to free key family members to do other things safe in the knowledge of the person being with someone
- use of technology to video call rather than having to travel to the hospital
- visitor books (physical and online) for family and friends to share observations with each other and updates on visits
- rotas to support visits, providing lifts and emotional support when having to leave hospital to go home
- Using technology to reduce feeling alone such as having heating and lighting that comes on at a certain time or can be switched on remotely so the family doesn't have to return home after visiting to dark and cold home
- Encouraging families to keep a collection of ready-to-eat foods in the bedside locker of the person (such as muesli/energy bars, nuts, fruit, noodles/soups) or in a hospital bag that they take to visit or have an emergency cash stash in their bags for the canteen to ensure that they do not neglect their own care whilst caring for the person
- Encouraging families to record a selection of: recounting a special memory, scripture readings, poems of significance, songs etc which can be played to the person when they cannot be present can be helpful

Involving families in sessions, practical discussions about discharge planning, and best interests decision-making can also provide subtle opportunities to investigate and promote self-care. Whilst it is important to offer specific space and time for families, 1:1, and as a whole family to consider their own needs, it is not unusual to hear them want the complete focus to be on the patient. Their assertion is typically that they cannot focus on themselves yet as all their emotional energy and headspace is taken up with the obvious and apparent needs of the profoundly injured family member. We have tended to find that families like to know that there are groups and resources we can signpost for them to use in our services, whether or not they choose to use these. We have found that they rarely want to attend peer support style groups arranged by staff, and instead prefer to develop their own peer relationships with families on the ward. Amongst those that do forge peer connections with other families struggling with similar issues, this can be a huge source of support, although conversely their different approaches to supporting the injured person can serve as real points of difference between them and become problematic. For example, when some partners have to return to work for financial necessity, other people's partners may view their lack of time visiting as indicative of a lack of connection with the injured person. Or, indeed if one person makes gains and progress whilst the other doesn't. At other times, we have seen that families will 'adopt' another patient and provide a conduit to the family who cannot be there as often by creating video calls and providing information. This is typically welcomed by families and seen as supportive but can be more challenging to negotiate for clinical staff who are legally, ethically, and morally tasked with ensuring the 'patient', who cannot give any form of valid consent for this apparent goodwill gesture, continues to have their confidentially and dignity protected by the services responsible for ensuring that. It can also be associated with risk when a family makes assumptions that the needs of the other patient are the same as their family member and can inadvertently respond by providing food or drink for example when that is not clinically indicated as safe. It is important that clinical teams are alert to these developing relationships.

Severe injuries have a way of resetting the networks around a person and can involve bringing back into a person's life family members who may have drifted away from regular contact or indeed been on the other side of a relational rupture before the injury. It can be difficult to understand what the person would have wanted for themselves in this context. Would bridges have been rebuilt? Would all have been resolvable? This minefield of human relationships requires great sensitivity and needs time. Members of the clinical team will inevitably have to try to grapple with the issues and the strong feelings of all involved. We recall having a man with a profound traumatic brain injury admitted, and over the following days, we met the mother of his children, his ex-wife, his current wife, his current girlfriend, and his work colleague with whom he had been sporadically romantically connected . As Valentine's day approached, this network of women who all had strong and caring feelings toward him were dropping off thoughtful gifts and cards filled with sentiment and slowly became aware of the existence of each other. They all seemed to consider that they were the primary carer, we should liaise with them only, and that the others should be barred from visiting. They all began to try to set up their own control over the others by being present by his bedside at all times. He was totally unable to guide what he wanted the clinical staff to do as he was unaware and unable to understand the complexities of the situation, and the clinical staff were left trying to establish a management plan that worked for him and supported his networks. We took the opinion that he had a legal wife we needed to clinically liaise with, but that he had apparently been connected to all the women; he had balanced a way to be with all of them at the same time and we needed to assist his recovery by ensuring people that were important to him remained involved in his life. We stopped the tearing down of items the last visitor had papered his walls with in favour of the new visitor's items by reminding all that holding his needs central was required. He had, whatever they all felt about the rights and wrongs of it, seen the value of being involved in all their lives. He had cognitive needs for controlled levels of visual/perceptual stimulation and reduced sensory overload. We brokered a deal that all could have photos in albums that they showed him on their own visit, but that the only permanent photos on the wall were those of each of his children. Families have unique dynamics and complexities that clinical teams need to gain a rapid appreciation of, to ensure sensitivity and problem-solving skills whilst keeping the patient at the centre of best interests decision-making.

Most family members develop their own understandings of the person's situation and future at their own speed. Some families will be on the same page, but others may not even be in the same chapter or even the same book! It is common to find differences between people's perspectives in the same family, with strong beliefs and feelings about what should be done, what is in the person's best interests, and this has the potential for further familial divides, distress, and conflict. It is quite common that the injury will spark a renegotiation of roles in the networks, including who will spend the most time at the bedside and who will feel they should have the most say in decisions about the person's life. Parents of adults with brain injury may become far more involved in their life again, spouses may be pulled in multiple directions with other demands (such as work, finances, and childcare responsibilities), children may be fearful or bored of visiting and refuse, some family members may find it too painful and difficult to visit and stop. These changes to roles and relationships all have the potential for familial distress and conflict. It is important to hold in mind as teams that the less frequent visitors do not care less, mean less to the person, or should have less weight given to their views. They may for example be more resigned to the diagnosis and accepting of the prognosis, whilst the daily bedside visitor remains hopeful and optimistic for further gains. It doesn't mean that one of them cares more than the other – they just have different perspectives on what this caring means.

Given that the family all had unique, personal, and different preinjury relationships with the person (such as spouse, favourite sibling, less in common sibling, parent, child, best friend, secret lover, co-worker, etc), it is natural that they will all have unique responses to the impact of the injury on themselves and what they want for the person. It can be helpful for them to notice and acknowledge this. In our work, sharing the adage 'we are in the same storm but in different boats' can be a helpful way to begin to discuss this.

Klonoff (2010) described the need to increase family members' awareness of the person with brain injury's post-injury strengths and their limitations, accept the new reality and identity, and be realistic, as principles to help family well-being and prevent unrealistic optimism. Some family members will show great desire to be involved in neurorehabilitation and derive optimism and foster ongoing hope for recovery through seeing gains, however small, in clinical sessions (such as being able to see the tilt table has moved another 10 degrees) and becoming trained to deliver stretches. Others appear to derive connectedness through caring tasks, such as involvement in washing, dressing, and grooming. Others take lead roles in preparing favourite music playlists and decorating the bed space with items and photos of important life events. We also see family members who seek to advocate, challenge the clinicians, confront the status quo, seek more input, and more time to drive neurorehabilitation. However family members approach things, this is a process that is not simple and takes time.

Complex neuro-disability is life-long. For families, they are challenged to learn to live with and cope with something that they cannot change or achieve substantial change in. For families who care for the person with such catastrophic brain injury, this can create a grief with no end. Olshansky termed this 'chronic sorrow', a normal response to the pain and devastation of living with the losses created by the injury and stemming from the disparity of the life imagined with the reality of the life as it is now (Klonoff et al., 2017).

Staff are often concerned by family members who are very distressed and flag these people to psychologists for support but can equally be concerned about families who appear to be 'in denial' and who do not appear to be expressing signs of grief. Our research has indicated that many healthcare staff hold unhelpful understandings and historical models of loss from other areas of life experience and erroneously apply these to the complex neuro-disability world. Post-modern theories of grief such as the dual processing model (Stroebe & Schut, 1999) highlight that the family members are in oscillation between restorative activities (attending to life changes) and loss-orientated activities (experiencing the intrusion of grief). Supporting families and staff to understand the experience of oscillating between loss-orientated moments and restorative activities is normal and can be helpful.

As clinical neuropsychologists, our work with families involves holding a sufficiently safe therapeutic space to allow families to say the unsayable and wonder aloud things like, *'would it have been better if she had died?'* and how their own role in the journey may have contributed to the reality of now *'we fought with the doctors in ICU to keep him alive, I think we did* the wrong thing', 'any part of her is better than being dead, we have to have hope', and grappling with the beliefs they hold about what the person themselves would have been likely to say about their own situation *'there's just no way she would have thought this was living'*. Families have already dealt with the earliest days of great uncertainty in the injury management, where the focus is on life-sustaining treatment, and it is less clear which patients will do better. Families tend to, by necessity in the face of overwhelmed coping resources, live moment to moment but with an expectation that the end point will be better than this. Discussions with clinical neuropsychologists to help families begin to look forward and consider the future are particularly critical when a person is in PDOC and decisions about the futility of treatment and a person's best interests (Mental Capacity Act 2005) legally need discussion. These conversations are very difficult and painful for families and often are said 1:1 with staff as when they are in a family group this can feel too exposing and treacherous.

Families faced with PDOC are in a unique, abnormal, and deeply distressing situation and cope in a variety of ways (Kitzinger & Kitzinger, 2014). Families experience complex distress (Soeterik et al., 2017) and grapple to find new roles and ways of still being together in the changed family system. Soeterik et al. (2018) found a unique form of Ambiguous Loss (Boss, 2000) in research with families of people in PDOC. Ambiguous loss creates a 'goodbye without leaving' where the person is alive and physically present but is no longer accessible to the family (psychologically absent). Soeterik et al. (2018) described how the loss caused by the brain injury was not easily addressed by families' own pre-existing understandings of loss, as there was no death. Their relationships were so fundamentally altered by the brain injury. Relationships were now hard to label by conventional titles, and families tended to be frozen, unable to look forward as it was too scary and unable to look back as it was too painful to remember (Soeterik et al., 2018). For clinical neuropsychologists approaching this work, psychological support should involve demonstrating a sensitivity to this unique complex loss, a validation of the losses, a framework for naming the loss, provision of education about the condition to help make sense of it, and ways to enhance coping with a chronic situation.

PDOC also creates unique issues in staff-family relationships (Chinner et al., 2022). Whilst healthcare professionals are meeting the person for the first time post-injury and considering what disability management needs they may have to maintain, improve, and prevent deterioration (such as splinting and getting a person seated) which will have wider benefits for the person (such as reducing pain, enabling digestion, access to a range of environments) and enable the person's brain to make whatever recovery it can, the family is contemplating what has been 'lost' from the person they knew and what must be regained. This difference in approach sets up from the start a potential for conflict – families are expecting staff to do something to help the person recover, and staff are trying to maximise the setting for the person's brain and prevent physical decline. Research has indicated that PDOC family members can feel symbiotically connected to the person (Soeterik et al., 2018) and talk in terms of 'we' (ie we had pneumonia last week). Thus, the roller coaster of medical instability of person in PDOC is also ridden by the family. This can mean that an inevitable decrease of direct input for the person in PDOC is similarly experienced by the family and can feel to them like abandonment. Whilst staff may erroneously consider that the family are struggling to cope with the one event (the injury), the reality for families is that they describe multiple life-threatening events (such as near loss due to infections, surgeries and having been called in to say goodbye multiple times already) as well as interactions with family, friends, and staff that can be distressing for them. Being aware of a trauma-informed approach (Ranjbar & Erb, 2019) to working with families is as crucially important as understanding this in relation to patients.

Whilst a gross oversimplification, we do see several types of common familial responses to such severe and complex neuro-disability:

- Those who accept at face value that the world has changed and become deeply invested in getting to know the new person post-injury want to be closely involved on a day-to-day basis
- Those who continue to strive, advocate, and seek for therapies and actions to help recover the old pre-injury person or who await a 'miracle' intervention
- Those who decide that the person is so fundamentally changed that the relationship is now so altered, their relationship is unrecognisable with the person and no longer meets their mutual needs, so the relationship ends (divorces may occur and visiting may cease)
- Those who wish to remain peripherally involved, ensure the person's care and life is optimised and inform decision-making, but no longer are as integrated in the day-to-day issues of their life (and indeed may form new romantic relationships externally, but wish to continue to remain married to the person with the brain injury)
- Those who decide that the injury has devastated the person's life but that they must now prioritise minimising the destruction of others' lives (e.g. children) and focus on the wider family

We recommended sharing that we have seen families take a wide variety of approaches to cope with the situation they find themselves in and take an overtly agnostic view on what individual family members may consider to be best for themselves. Whatever decision people take, it is usually very painful and requires significant renegotiation with the wider familial network who will have their own opinions about it.

When people are discharged from the service, this can be a real point of challenge for families. Discharge is often representative of a growing awareness that all the changes that they had hoped for have not been able to happen. For some families, the totality and the future for their family comes into stark reality. Families are faced with managing choices about the 'best' specialist centre or the 'closest' location to them. It is important for clinicians to help families to consider that not everything that is known about managing complex brain injury must be tried in this setting, at this time. The rehabilitation journey is long, and different aspects of neurorehabilitation may have different prominence at different time points. It is helpful to focus on the stage of the person's journey that you join them for and the priorities for that stage. As and when people make gains and changes, then services allow for a revolving door to enable a further targeted rehabilitative effort.

References

Boss, P. (2000). Ambiguous Loss: Learning to Live with Unresolved Grief. Harvard University Press

Chinner, A., Pauli, R., & Cruse, D. (2022). The impact of prolonged disorders of consciousness on family caregivers' quality of life – A scoping review. *Neuropsychological Rehabilitation, 32*(7), 1643–1666. https://doi.org/10.1080/09602011.2021.1922463

Kitzinger, C., & Kitzinger, J. (2014). Grief, anger and despair in relatives of severely brain injured patients: Responding without pathologising. *Clinical Rehabilitation, 28*(7), 627–631.

Klonoff, P. S. (2010). Psychotherapy for Families After Brain Injury: Principles and Techniques. New York: Guildford Press.

Klonoff, P. S., Strang. B., & Perumparaichallai, K. (2017). Family-based support for people with brain injury. In Neuropsychological Rehabilitation. The International Handbook. B.A. Wilson, J. Winegardner, C. M. Heugten and T. Ownsworth (Eds), pp. 364–777.

Ranjbar, N., & Erb, M. (2019). Adverse childhood experiences and trauma-informed care in rehabilitation clinical practice. *Archives of Rehabilitation Research and Clinical Translation, 1*, 1–2. https://doi.org/10.1016/j.arrct.2019.100003.

Smith, D & Worthington, A. (2024). A legal framework for the management of challenging behaviour. In Managing Challenging Behaviour Following Acquired Brain Injury Assessment, Intervention and Measuring Outcomes. N. Alderman & A. Worthington (Eds). Routledge.

Soeterik, S. M., Connolly, S., Playford, E. D., Duport, S., & Riazi, A. (2017). The psychological impact of prolonged disorders of consciousness on caregivers: A systematic review of quantitative studies. *Clinical Rehabilitation, 31*(10), 1374–1385.

Soeterik, S. M., Connolly, S., & Riazi, A. (2018). "Neither a wife nor a widow": an interpretative phenomenological analysis of the experiences of female family caregivers in disorders of consciousness. *Neuropsychological Rehabilitation, 28*(8), 1392–1407.

Stroebe, M., & Schut, H. (1999). The dual process model of coping with bereavement: Rationale and description. *Death Studies, 23*(3), 197–224. https://doi.org/10.1080/074811899201046

11 Effective teamworking in complex neuro-disability

Throughout the chapters in this book, you will have seen references to teamwork and the importance of neurorehabilitative efforts being collaborative. There is a consensus that the aims of neurorehabilitation are to enable a person to reach their maximum potential across a range of functions and manage things that cannot improve to prevent complications and deterioration through disability management. Given the complexities of a person's neuro-disabilities, there is a clear necessity and understanding that neurorehabilitation will need a team comprising professionals from a range of different clinical disciplines. The following box shows the range of those commonly involved in addition to a person's family.

Professions who might be involved in brain injury rehabilitation alongside the family

Clinical neuropsychology	Physiotherapy	Occupational therapy
Rehabilitation nursing	Speech and language therapy	Rehabilitation medicine
Neuropsychiatry	Social work	Dietitians
Tissue viability nurse	Continence nurses	ITU nurses
Fresenius nurses	Healthcare assistants	Specialist brain injury support workers
Music therapy	Art therapy	Specialist dentistry
Wheelchair/seating specialists	Equipment specialists	Assistive technology specialists
Vocational specialists	Benefits advisors	Neurosurgeons
Housing advisors	Case management	Third-sector providers like Headway groups

(Continued)

DOI: 10.4324/9781032665986-11

Professions who might be involved in brain injury rehabilitation alongside the family

---

Podiatrists/chiropodists	Therapy/psychology assistants	Neuro-ophthalmologists
Neurologists	Audiovestibular consultants	Orthopaedic consultants
Respiratory physicians	ENT consultants	Postural management specialists
Clinical psychologists	Admission/discharge coordinators	Pharmacists
Educational psychologists	Faith/community leaders	Learning support advisors

Whilst this may seem like a large list, it should be remembered that this is not an exhaustive list. There are likely to be other specialists involved where a person has comorbidities such as diabetes, epilepsy, neuroendocrinology needs, and so on. It is unlikely that all these people will be involved at the same time, with who is involved gradually evolving as the person progresses from acute care through to long-term care. Of course, some of this huge team do remain involved throughout, such as the family, and this is important to consider in terms of leadership and team dynamics. When there are so many different neurorehabilitation collaborators involved, how these people work together is of paramount importance.

Whilst neurorehabilitation and complex disability management are important, there are a number of challenges in delivering this. The following box sets out a selection of common clinical conundrums that are faced in teamwork.

Common clinical conundrums in teamwork

When many team members are involved, the timetable gets filled, and the patient's fatigue levels interfere with progress

Setting up processes to manage the team rather than the needs of the people we work with, e.g. documentation that reflects funders' demands rather than the way the team works

Just because you can do it doesn't mean you should, or that you should do it now

Forgetting the bigger picture

Common clinical conundrums in teamwork

Time for supervision and reflection is not a luxury; it is a fundamental
    requirement for good teamwork with this group
Avoid 'group think', a bias that can develop from an attempt to
    create harmony or consensus even when the evidence is poor for
    that consensus, resulting in poor decision-making
Not managing professional boundaries

11.1 Creating a team

Creating a team is not as simple as bringing a group of different professionals
together (Singh et al., 2018). It requires shared aims, a respect for and
understanding of the contributions made by other team members and an
ability to work in collaboration with others to achieve shared goals. If this is
achieved, then teamwork becomes extremely powerful with the outcomes
from the team being greater than what might be achieved by the team
members working in a unidisciplinary fashion. However, teams in most
neurorehabilitation settings evolve rather than staff being recruited specifically to join the team. Clinicians rotate through the organisation to be in
the team or are generally allocated by professional leads or case managers
based on the needs of departments, systems, and/or previous relationships
with the clinician. How a team operates is heavily influenced, if not entirely
determined, by wider organisational demands. For example, therapy is
usually contractually agreed for a time-limited period by the funders, and
the structure of a programme will be influenced by this with goal setting,
reporting, timings of various meetings, and work set to meet this externally
imposed contracted timetable, rather than led by the needs of the patient or
their family. Creating a 'team culture' therefore depends on the leadership of
the team, the paperwork and processes that support the team, and a shared
understanding of the team ethos, purpose, and formulation.

From the outset, the team will all be appraising the growing mass of data
and information about a person and trying to work from it. In complex neuro-
disability, this requires a lot of communication, and managing this is difficult. Seeking on the one hand to work efficiently and not involve everyone
in everything, and on the other hand to be able to zoom out and look at
the bigger picture, checking for patterns and trends. Supporting the family,
who believe that no stone should be left unturned, whilst at the same time
appeasing managers, who frequently do not understand the importance of the
time the team spends in discussion and planning, is a difficult path to tread. It
is also crucial to ensure that the time spent in meetings is used efficiently and
profitably for the patient.

In order to create a team culture and to discuss, build, and share formulations about a person's presentation, the team must have dedicated and protected time to meet. Meetings are needed to consider planning, formulating, goal setting, feeding back, and reflecting on how challenges were met and how they might be best tackled in the future. In contrast, others can view this indirect work about a patient as problematic. Allocating time to do this properly is nearly always a mission because at a management level there remains a view that unless a clinician has a patient in front of them, they are not doing their job. This is largely a hangover of management from within a medical model, where the expectation was that therapists were given instructions by medical consultants, and no shared formulation was attempted.

For a team to work efficiently and deliver the best rehabilitation programmes, it is necessary for them to have paperwork that supports the way that they work. Often paperwork is imposed by organisations or funders, but without the understanding of how complex neuro-disability may not fit this. There is an expectation that work will proceed through a process of a patient identifying their priorities and goals for rehabilitation and collaboratively setting goals with their team, and that these goals should be SMART goals. Whilst this is certainly important in many aspects of neurorehabilitation, it does not necessarily reflect working with this cohort of complex neuro-disability patients (see Chapter 3), when a person cannot contribute to the planning of their rehabilitation and setting goals with the patient may not be possible at all. If goals are set, they are usually set by the clinical team. Where this is the case, the principle of best interests decision-making is needed (as the person is not able to consent to the care and treatment being recommended), and then it becomes even more important that the team focuses not on what they can do for a patient, but on what the person might choose to do, including where they might choose to stop.

There is a tendency to think of good goal planning as involving only a few goals at a time, with additional goals added as achieved goals occur. Planning and prioritising the order of interventions is a matter that needs to be considered at a team level because all goals are not equal in terms of the demands that may be made on the brain-injured person. Consider the difference between working on a showering goal versus working on a continence goal. The process of showering is likely to be longer and involve more stages, and the person is likely to require a rest at the end of the task. Visiting the toilet by comparison is likely to be shorter and generally will not require a rest period following each visit to the toilet. However, going to the toilet happens multiple times a day and engaging with the physical and cognitive demands to focus on this goal runs right throughout the day, and it is likely that a person will experience higher levels of fatigue and possibly associated irritability when this is begun. Trying to work on other goals is likely to be more difficult when working on continence, and adjustments should therefore be made at these times. Clearly, this requires some coordination and cooperation across the team, and to achieve this, the demands of the different interventions must be understood by the whole team, and the timing of such must be agreed. It may be appealing to have rules about how many goals a person is working on at any one time, but this does not work well in practice.

How a team works out these priorities depends on the needs of the person they are working with at that time. However, there are likely to be challenges and conflicts within teams. In a study by van der Veen et al. (2024), they considered what facilitates and impedes team functioning in a neurorehabilitation team, focusing on team identification, psychological safety, and team learning. The results of their study revealed that a strong sense of team identity was not sufficient to ensure good team learning. Of great importance was a team's ability to engage in constructive conflict and develop 'a shared mental model'. In this context, we can describe this shared mental model as akin to a shared formulation. Engaging in constructive conflict demands a sense of psychological safety, and this is impacted by factors that have been previously identified as concerns about hierarchies within a team, the expectations of the team members' professional bodies, and the concept of clinical autonomy (van der Veen et al., 2024; O'Donovan & Mcauliffe (2020)).

11.2 Models of teamwork

In the neurorehabilitation literature, there are references to multidisciplinary, interdisciplinary, and transdisciplinary teamwork but what these terms actually mean is often poorly understood. Karol (2014) provides a helpful summary of the differences between these models of teamwork. Multidisciplinary teamwork (MDT) fits with a medical model approach to rehabilitation and is therefore led by a medic. These teams consist of a group of people from different disciplines with clearly demarcated roles. Karol (2014) described that the MDT 'carve up the person' by their areas of expertise, with no overlap between the disciplines. The person's rehabilitation needs are identified as problems, and these problems are addressed by the discipline claiming the part of the person into which that problem fits. Communication goes via the medical consultant, and goal setting is unidisciplinary rather than coordinated and collaborative.

Interdisciplinary teamwork does recognise the overlap between some clinical disciplines and allows for different areas of overlap. However, clinical issues are still assigned according to discipline. The areas of overlap create a necessity for the different disciplines to engage in more communication and usually result in better coordination of the rehabilitation programme. Karol (2014) comments about interdisciplinary working that, 'The model incorporates treatment plans, teaching approaches, educational initiatives, and interventions that are at least compatible and preferably similar'.

Transdisciplinary working encompasses a shift away from organising rehabilitation according to the expertise of different disciplines, instead taking the goals that the person with the brain injury is striving towards as the starting point and considering how each of the different disciplines can contribute to the person reaching these. It does *not* mean that everyone on the team is expected to undertake all the specialist roles, or do a bit of every therapy. For this approach to work, the whole team needs to share a formulation that describes the presentation of the individual and the aims/goals of the rehabilitation at that point. It is recognised that rehabilitation is an iterative process with ongoing assessment, hypothesis building and testing, intervention and reassessment and as such is dynamic and its aims/goals are expected to develop and change. This approach is particularly helpful for patients with complex neuro-disability who have complex needs. This requires a high level of communication and collaboration, and good leadership from a leader who understands the transdisciplinary approach and whom the team trusts.

Transdisciplinary working, as highlighted, is not all disciplines working on all things. The growth of the health and well-being industry within Western society in recent years has led to the popularisation of psychological terminology and awareness and the use of psychological techniques more generally. Associated with this has been a trend for team members without clinical neuropsychology training to bring this to their own work with patients, especially when there may not be a psychologist available. Arguably there are issues for teams to consider about staying within their scope of practice. This is critical in complex neuro-disability, where a fulsome understanding of emotional functioning and the cognitive and communication impairments is vital. Using a treatment method (such as a technique from ACT or CBT or mindfulness) requires an assessment of the underlying psychological need, a formulation of the broader issues and a clinical decision about the optimal psychological model to best understand the situation and evidence-based way to tackle this.

11.3 Team leadership

Leading a large and constantly evolving team inevitably involves keeping a lot of plates spinning. The patient is always the centre point of the programme and therefore must be the first consideration of the team leader. However, in order to ensure that a transdisciplinary approach is maintained, the team leader must also be aware of the needs and views of the different team members, the family and the funders, which at times will be competing. Different team members will approach the rehabilitation programme at different speeds, either because of the nature of their role, the urgency of what they are responding to, or the nature of their personality and competing priorities in their own workload. Those who have more task-based roles often find their work is faster paced than the work of team members whose roles are more process-based. Working at different paces can lead to friction between team members, especially when a patient has limited resources and/or high levels of fatigue and there is some competition for the 'windows' of rehabilitation opportunities.

An important role for the team leader is to take a holistic view of the needs of the brain-injured person and support the person, their family, and the team to understand that priorities for rehabilitation include consideration of what is most appropriate to work on in the current setting versus future settings. For example, some of an inpatient clinical team might insist that a patient's admission must be extended because they still have goals to work on. Inevitably, in the context of so much need, a person will always have ongoing goals that staff can help with. Judging the best location for these to be worked on effectively needs consideration (e.g. if someone is returning to a family home, working on a Sara Steady standing transfer from bed to the chair is best in the location where the skill will be needed). The broader issue of retaining a patient past a possible endpoint of the admission is that families can gain unrealistic expectations of significant further change and become highly frustrated that change is not occurring at the anticipated rate.

The role of the team leader must be to ensure that the contributions of all the members of the team add up to a symphony rather than a noise, as Prigatano (1999) described it. Who is best to fulfil this role will depend to some extent on the make-up of the team and the personalities within it. The person leading the team must have a good understanding of the roles and responsibilities of the team members involved. They must have a good overview of the needs of the patients treated by the teams, and they must understand the process of formulation in the context of neurorehabilitation. Historically, teams have been led by medical consultants because they hold the medical responsibility for the patient, but medics may have very little involvement in the process of rehabilitation as the person's medical stability increases, and the further away from the acute setting that a person moves. The team leader in a post-acute or community neurorehabilitation setting is increasingly the neuropsychologist, and this is usually because they have an understanding of team formulation, team dynamics, an appreciation of the roles of other professions, and an ability to hold the bigger picture in mind. In addition, they are often well suited to creating a sense of team identification and psychological safety which enables team members to challenge colleagues in a robust way without this feeling threatening.

Leadership requires managing rehabilitation priorities and making difficult decisions about what may and may not be helpful to continue to invest patient and staff time as well as resources on. For example, exploring cognitive function or communicative ability with a person in different settings (bed, wheelchair, standing frame etc) can be hugely informative. However, discovering that someone communicates best in a hydrotherapy pool, for example, may not be particularly functional, given they cannot spend hours in such a setting. The rewards of finding a positive behaviour need to be weighed against the utility of that behaviour and the cost of it in terms of energy and resources. Just because something is possible to achieve does not mean it is necessarily where rehabilitative efforts should be put. In an area where there is less positive feedback for therapists, it is very rewarding to make a change and very hard for therapists when the team seeks to focus efforts elsewhere. Managing challenges like this requires careful leadership.

Good leadership involves ensuring that all team members have a voice and that all team members feel that their roles are valued. Teams need to be free to have a sense of exploration and experimentation rather than dictation. Psychologists are specifically trained to manage groups and complex emotional situations and support or challenge risk to ensure that the least risky option is not always chosen, but rather that positive risk-taking and the most appropriate choice to further a person's rehabilitation are enabled. Supporting robust best interests decision-making within teams is often a role the neuropsychologist undertakes. These are some of the reasons that neuropsychologists often find themselves in leadership roles in teams, but these skills are not unique to neuropsychologists, and team leaders should be chosen on the basis of their skills rather than belonging to a specific discipline.

11.4 The process of rehabilitation and goal setting

The more complex the person's situation, the more people are likely to be involved in their care and rehabilitation, and the need for leadership, organisation, and containment becomes increasingly necessary. Prigatano (1999) describes this as careful orchestration. The people who are part of the team will be contributing very different aspects of care and rehabilitation. Some people have roles that are focused on tasks that need completing, and other people's roles are more focused on process. There are often questions remaining within the formulation, and there can be a tendency for some team members to see rehabilitation as serial steps, 'You sort out this matter and once you've done that I can then get on with this other matter', but rehabilitation is not serial; it needs to be conducted in parallel. For example, therapists don't wait to work on standing until wheelchair skills have been mastered. Similarly, the idea that challenging behaviour must be addressed before 'rehabilitation' can begin is not helpful. Managing concurrent rehabilitation in turn requires time and space for good communication so that change, or lack of it, can be considered in the context of different aspects of the programme and their influence on each other. The importance of a shared formulation is clear in this context because the different aspects of a biopsychosocial model all interact and are not simply a list of factors that need consideration in isolation. This requires organisation and prioritisation of the work of the team.

The basis of teamwork in this setting is first to identify behaviours that a person might exhibit, whether they are helpful or unhelpful, to assess what we are able to across the biopsychosocial model, build a formulation through drawing hypotheses and testing them in order to strengthen and shape the formulation, and develop interventions on the basis of this. This is an iterative process, and at each iteration, the team must manage different opinions and priorities. The usual pattern of neurorehabilitation is to seek to create a rehabilitation programme that is 'patient led'. To find out what the patient wants to achieve and then to set goals with the patient that enable a path towards the goal to be seen and adopted, and so that progress, or otherwise, can be measured and the goals adapted as necessary. This sounds logical and sensible, but it is difficult to achieve, and patients with complex neuro-disability throw some additional difficulties into the path.

Perhaps the most challenging to consider is goal setting. Many services suggest that the goals are set by the patients themselves. Sometimes this is true but, depending on the extent and nature of the brain injury, the makeup and time of the rehabilitation specialists, the pressure from funders, and the abilities of the team leader, may not be accurate. For example, if a patient sets a goal for themselves that the therapy staff consider to be unachievable at all or unachievable in the admission period, they are left in a quandary. Some team members will suggest that working on this is potentially helpful, as the patient's failure to meet an unachievable goal will increase insight for the patient; others will consider this as setting someone up to fail and therefore unethical, whilst others might take the view that irrespective of if it is ethical or not, the patient will not be able to learn from failure. With complex neuro-disability, the dilemma goes a step further; the person is unlikely to be able to engage in goal setting in any meaningful way at all. So how should the team build a patient-centred rehabilitation programme?

In complex neuro-disability, a significant amount of the work to be done is not on promoting change or recovery but rather on managing the disabilities in order that they do not worsen. By maximising a patient's disability management, it enables the opportunity to assess what might be possible if, for example, better posture and breath control are achieved. Very often it is the management of pain, infection, posture, tone, skin, and so on that must be the starting point. These matters may require data gathering and hypothesis testing, but arguably they are not patient goals but rather actions selected and undertaken by the treating team.

One thing that is frequently observed by families and friends of the person with the brain injury is that their world is fundamentally different from pre-injury, and they want to know what is being done to regain this old life. It can be helpful to reflect on this and to consider the initial planning of a rehabilitation programme within this new and smaller world. This is likely to be useful in the initial stages of rehabilitation, where, whilst holding knowledge of the person's past achievements, joys and sadnesses, hopes and dreams, the steps that can be realistically approached, observed, and measured are made. This enables families to see a sense of movement or change.

11.5 The role of the neuropsychologist in the team

Within our direct work with patients, we gain a great deal of knowledge for the team from structured behavioural observations made within other clinicians' sessions. Observing others' sessions is an active process. We've made a decision to carry out observations within the setting of their therapy session to inform our assessment and formulation. This is because it is possible to infer so much about cognition, emotion, and behaviour from watching the inter-action, what they say, what they do, and how they cope with challenge.

Observation in other clinicians' session is distinct from joint sessions in which both parties are active in planning and carrying out the session task. These joint sessions need to be carefully planned, and the aims of the sessions considered and discussed ahead of the session taking place. For example, with speech and language therapists, we might do joint sessions to explore a person's ability to consistently and reliably use yes/no responses, make choices and explore their functional communication capacity, and conduct joint capacity assessments. With occupational therapists, we may design a multi-errands task together to explore cognition in function. We look at the impact of impaired cognition and anxiety within physical therapy sessions whilst trying out strategies like breathing or distraction etc.

For those who are unsure what to do with patients with complex neuro-disability, joint sessions can be a way to feel or look like you are doing some-thing when you don't know what to do. Obviously, this is in no one's best interests, and supervision and reflection will help with clinical reasoning to explore whether they have a role at that time, their own feelings of 'being stuck,' and a way to plan the next steps.

It is also the case that when there is little feedback from a patient, the ther-apist may well fill the gap themselves. The voicing of an assumption about a behaviour or the lack of a behaviour by one person can lead to that assumption being taken up by others in the team and 'group think' begins. This can be quite destructive to a rehabilitation programme. Neuropsychologists are good at spotting and challenging this problem because their role involves both the detail (e.g. of cognitive assessment or behavioural analysis) and zooming out to the bigger picture.

Integrating information from the family is a significant role for the neuro-psychologist, along with ensuring that the family is supported and the needs and views of all the family members are considered as plans for further inter-vention or placement are made.

It is recognised that working with this group of people is difficult and emo-tionally demanding. There is very limited direct feedback from the person with neuro-disability themselves. This can take its toll on the team members. It is important to try to prevent burnout and manage the sadness that team members often feel. The neuropsychologists on the team have a role in first-aiding members of the team and helping them to manage the very significant personal demands made on them, both for their own sakes and to ensure that the team can keep functioning. This is an interesting but difficult path to tread, as the psychologist needs to be part of the team but in this role is fulfilling a 'meta' function. It highlights the absolute need for good supervision and an opportunity for the psychologist to also seek out support to prevent burnout.

References

Karol, R. L. (2014). Team models in neurorehabilitation: Structure, function, and culture change. *NeuroRehabilitation, 34*(4), 655–669. https://doi.org/10.3233/NRE-141080

O'Donovan, R., & Mcauliffe, E. (2020). A systematic review of factors that enable psychological safety in healthcare teams. *International Journal for Quality in Health Care, 32*(4), 240–250. https://doi.org/10.1093/intqhc/mzaa025

Prigatano, G. P. (1999). Principles of Neuropsychological Rehabilitation. Oxford University Press.

Singh, R., Küçükdeveci, A. A., Grabljevec, K., & Gray, A. (2018). The role of interdisciplinary teams in physical and rehabilitation medicine. *Journal of Rehabilitation Medicine, 50*(8), 673–678. https://doi.org/10.2340/16501977-2364

van der Veen, R., van der Burgt, S., Königs, M., Oosterlaan, J., & Peerdeman, S. (2024). Team functioning in neurorehabilitation: A mixed methods study. *Journal of Interprofessional Care, 38*(4), 621–631. https://doi.org/10.1080/13561820.2024.2325694

Afterword

Most clinicians will not have had much direct experience of working with people with this level of complex neuro-disability. Yet, this clinical population is now growing in western cultures, and more clinicians will need to have the necessary knowledge and skills to support these patients. This is a clinical area filled with overwhelming levels of impairment. There is an absence of a suitable descriptor to categorise this level of catastrophic and profound outcome following a severe brain injury. Terms within this area are interpreted differently, usually according to a clinician's lack of exposure to the most devastating levels of neuro-disability. This cohort of patients are rarely able to make their own decisions and provide consent for assessment and treatment, leaving the professionals in their lives to hold great responsibility in determining what is done for them in their best interests. Discharging this duty of care to a patient requires the professional to have a strong understanding of the core issues faced by this population and their families.

Approaching assessment and rehabilitation for these patients is different, and even experienced clinicians can feel deskilled. When new to something, there is a tendency to reach for a manual to guide you or fall back on previous experience. However, in complex neuro-disability, there is no manual and past practice is usually not a helpful guide. The evidence base is limited and typically excludes the very people you are trying to find the evidence to help. The best advice is to stop and really think. This work requires a paradigm shift from the standard practice of seeing the person as largely intact with some areas of difficulty, to move to looking for any ability in the context of overwhelming impairment. Finding ability requires a return to first principles and to think about what you're trying to find out. Begin the search by looking at what a person can do and problem solve how to use this by establishing and using consistent and reproducible methods. You need to think not only about what you are trying to address but also how you might get to it. This is the scientist–practitioner method in action and relies on concepts familiar to you such as single case experimental design, reproducibility, reliability, and consistency.

What constitutes rehabilitation in the spectrum of complex neuro-disability is also different. By necessity it has both a high degree of disability management focus alongside varying levels of active neurorehabilitation. Formulation in this context involves bringing together the views of the family, who have a detailed understanding of the person but almost always have a limited understanding of the impact of the injury and recovery trajectory, with the views of the professionals, who better understand the injury and expected recovery trajectory, but who lack a sense of the person. Rarely is the person themselves able to contribute to any goal setting or guide the intervention. The absence of the person's own voice in neurorehabilitation puts additional pressures on the professionals to hold the person in mind and at the centre of all decision-making. It is important to focus in on the person's known values, wishes, and beliefs to help guide decision-making about their best interests and guide the rehabilitation plan more broadly. Where possible gaining an appreciation of the person's values and aspirations with them directly or through their families and naturalistic support networks is vital.

We hope this book has equipped practitioners with a mental framework to approach this important and challenging work.

Sonja, Sal, and Sarah

Index

For Product Safety Concerns and Information please contact our EU
representative GPSR@taylorandfrancis.com
Taylor & Francis Verlag GmbH, Kaufingerstraße 24, 80331 München, Germany

www.ingramcontent.com/pod-product-compliance
Lightning Source LLC
Chambersburg PA
CBHW060449240326
41598CB00088B/4255

* 9 7 8 1 0 3 2 6 6 5 9 3 1 *